AF824433

It's easy to get lost in the cancer world

Let NCCN Guidelines for Patients® be your guide

- ✓ Step-by-step guides to the cancer care options likely to have the best results
- ✓ Based on treatment guidelines used by health care providers worldwide
- ✓ Designed to help you discuss cancer treatment with your doctors

National Comprehensive Cancer Network®

NCCN Guidelines for Patients® are developed by the National Comprehensive Cancer Network® (NCCN®)

NCCN

- ✓ An alliance of leading cancer centers across the United States devoted to patient care, research, and education

Cancer centers that are part of NCCN:
NCCN.org/cancercenters

NCCN Clinical Practice Guidelines in Oncology (NCCN Guidelines®)

- ✓ Developed by doctors from NCCN cancer centers using the latest research and years of experience
- ✓ For providers of cancer care all over the world
- ✓ Expert recommendations for cancer screening, diagnosis, and treatment

Free online at
NCCN.org/guidelines

NCCN Guidelines for Patients

- ✓ Present information from the NCCN Guidelines in an easy-to-learn format
- ✓ For people with cancer and those who support them
- ✓ Explain the cancer care options likely to have the best results

Free online at
NCCN.org/patientguidelines

These NCCN Guidelines for Patients are based on the NCCN Guidelines® for T-Cell Lymphomas, Version 1.2022 — December 22, 2021

NCCN Foundation seeks to support the millions of patients and their families affected by a cancer diagnosis by funding and distributing NCCN Guidelines for Patients. NCCN Foundation is also committed to advancing cancer treatment by funding the nation's promising doctors at the center of innovation in cancer research. For more details and the full library of patient and caregiver resources, visit NCCN.org/patients.

National Comprehensive Cancer Network (NCCN) / NCCN Foundation
3025 Chemical Road, Suite 100
Plymouth Meeting, PA 19462
215.690.0300

NCCN Guidelines for Patients are supported by funding from the NCCN Foundation®

To make a gift or learn more, please visit NCCNFoundation.org/donate
or e-mail PatientGuidelines@NCCN.org.

With generous support from:

Erin K. Frantz
Marilyn and James L. Mohler, MD
Warren Smedley

Endorsed by The Leukemia & Lymphoma Society

The Leukemia & Lymphoma Society (LLS) is dedicated to developing better outcomes for blood cancer patients and their families through research, education, support and advocacy and is happy to have this comprehensive resource available to patients. lls.org/patientsupport

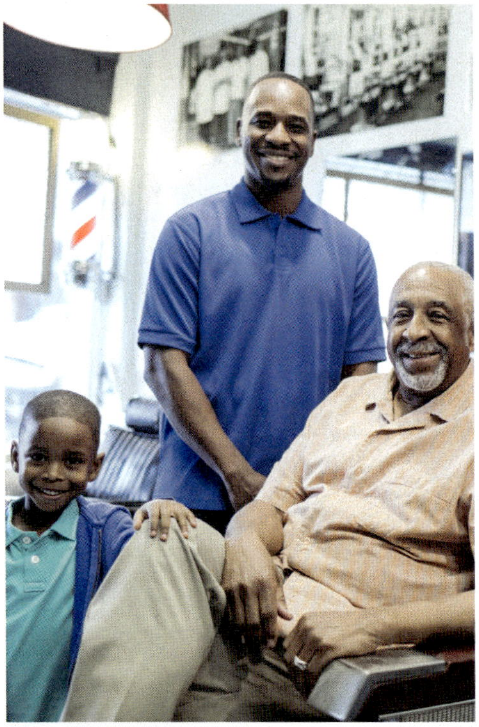
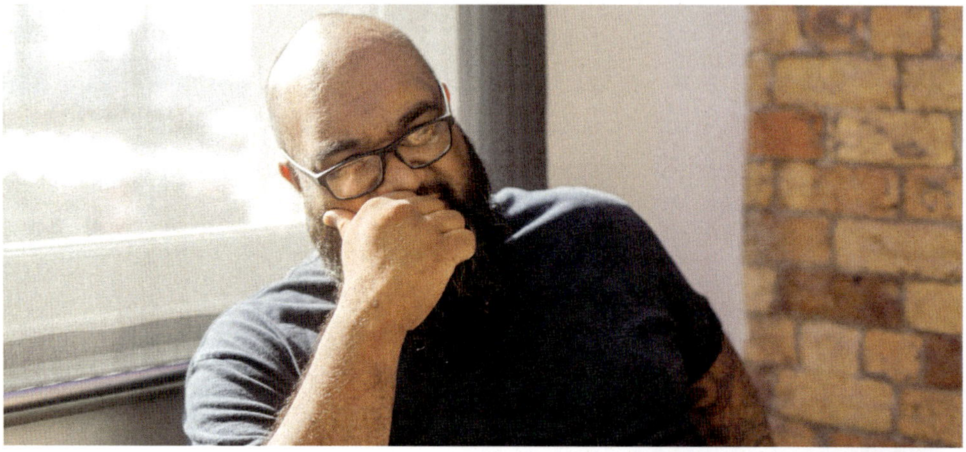
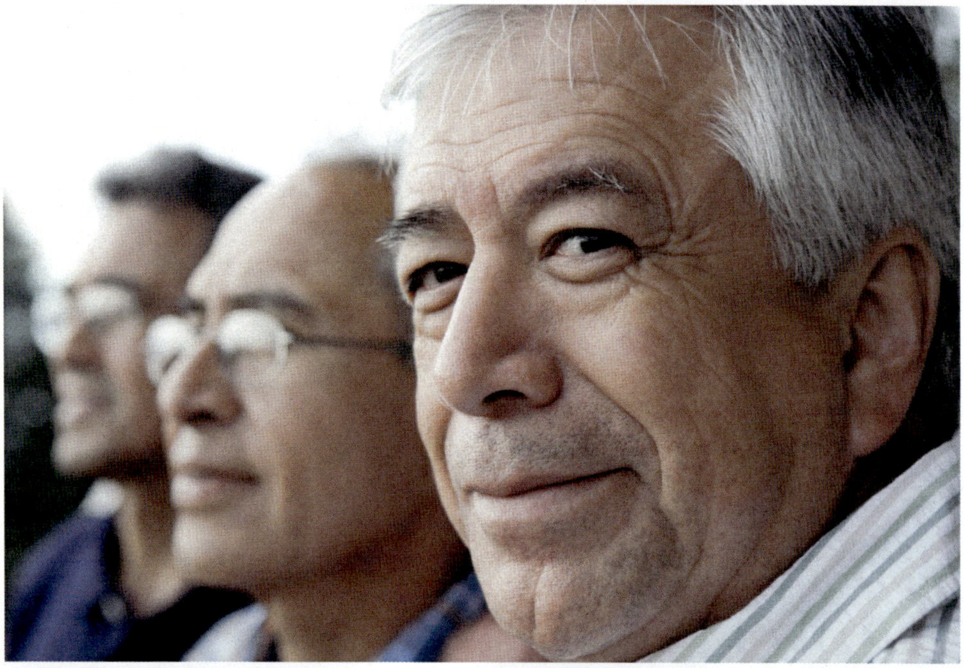
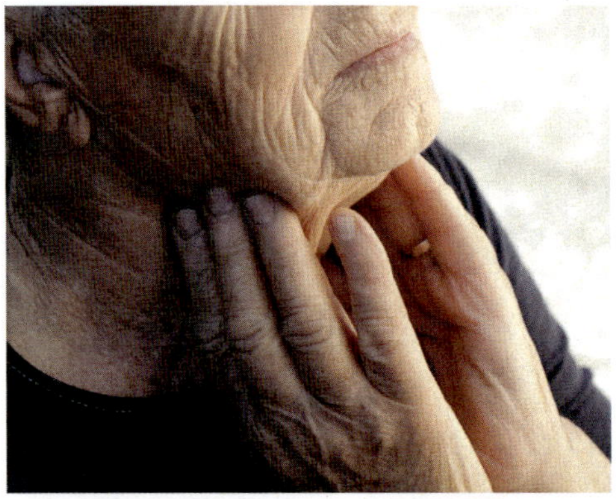
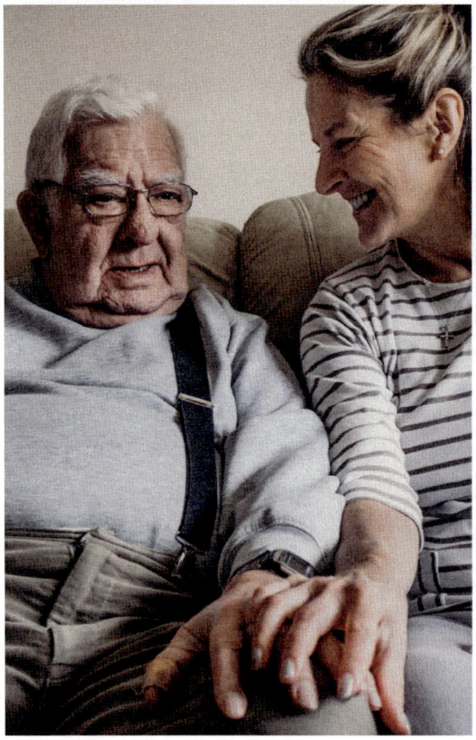
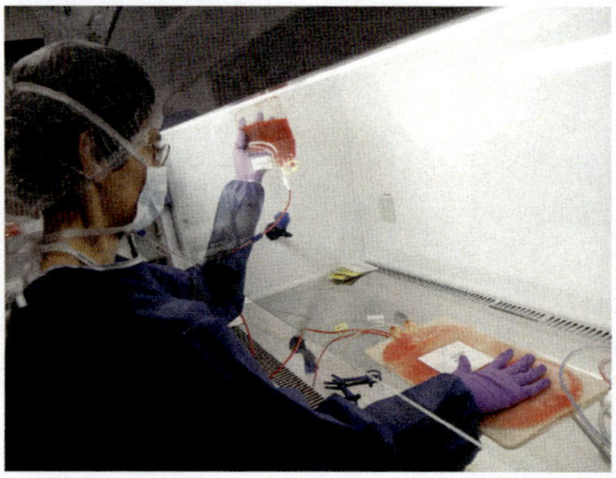
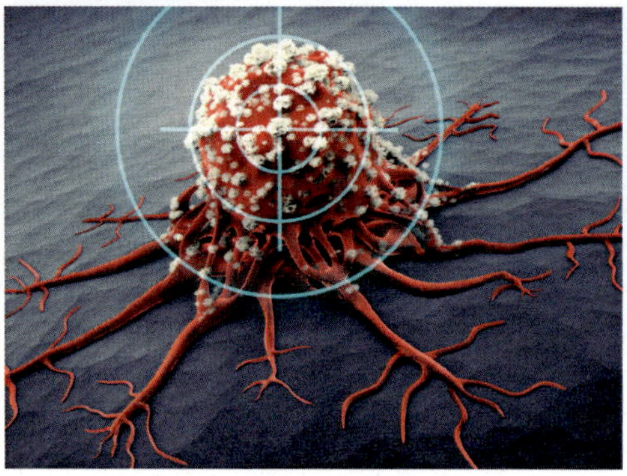
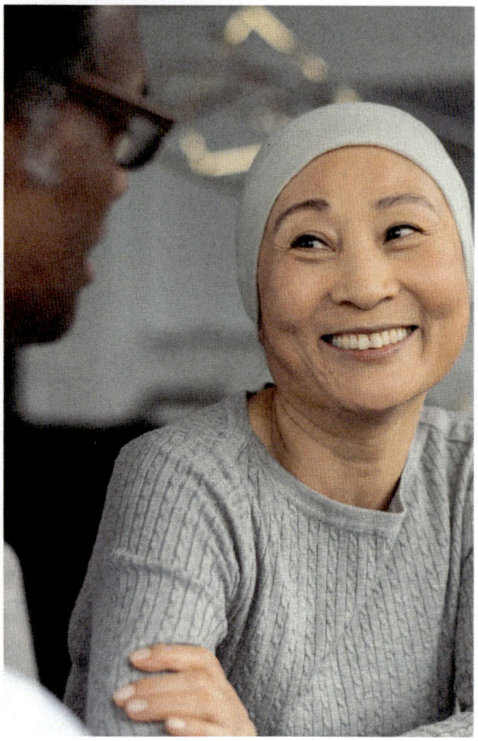

Contents

1 Peripheral T-cell lymphoma basics

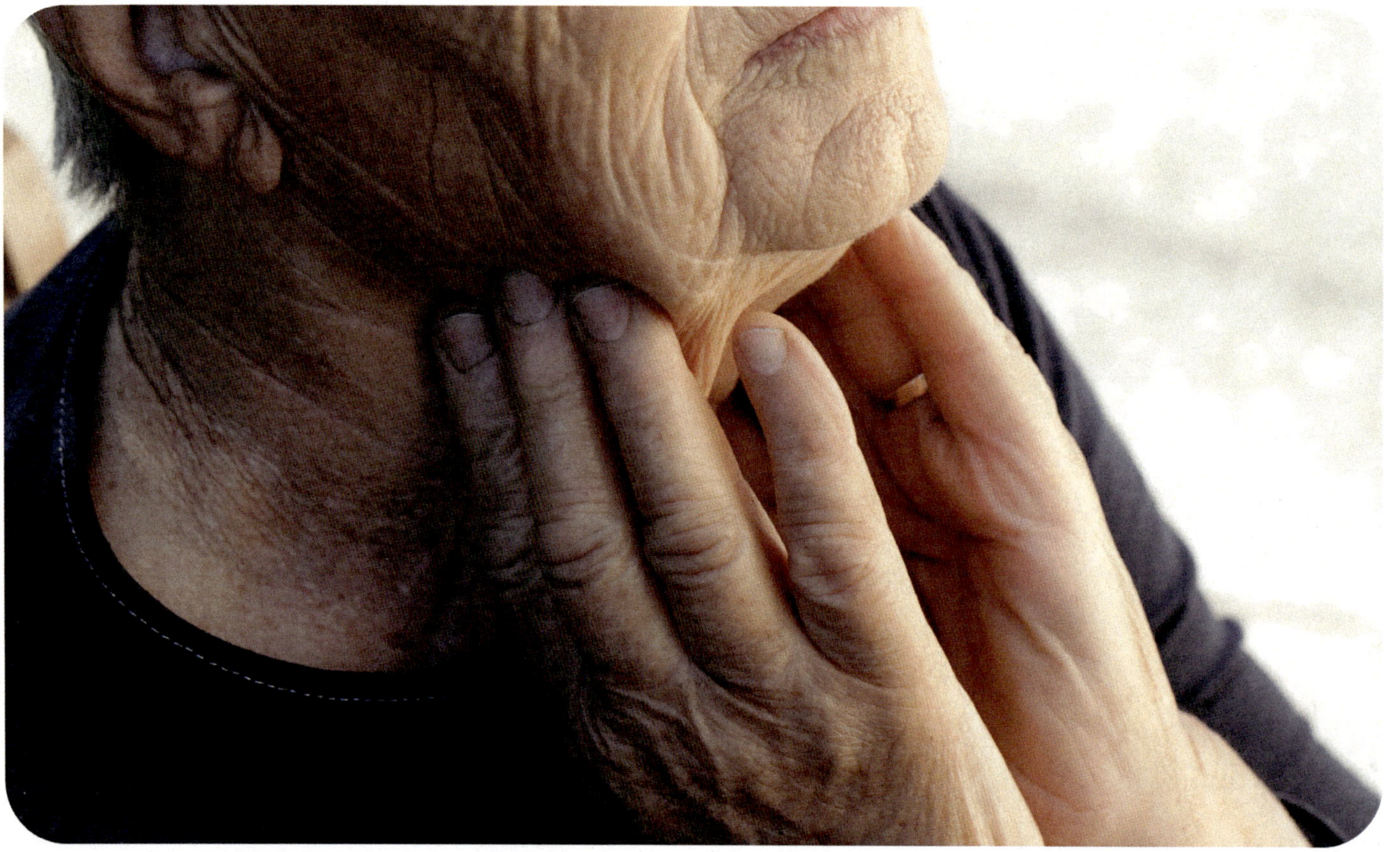

This chapter gives a short overview of peripheral T-cell lymphoma. You'll learn what it is, how it develops, what tests can diagnose it, and what can be done to treat it.

What is peripheral T-cell lymphoma?

Peripheral T-cell lymphoma is a rare cancer that's not easy to understand at first. It doesn't attack a single organ, such as in lung cancer or stomach cancer. Unlike those cancers, a lymphoma develops from certain blood cells and can grow anywhere in the body.

So what is it exactly?

Let's break it down word by word, from the last word to the first:

- **Lymphoma** – A lymphoma is a cancer in the lymphatic system. The lymphatic system is part of the immune system—the body's germ-fighting network. The lymphatic system includes the lymph nodes, spleen, gastrointestinal tract, and skin. A lymphoma is a type of blood cancer that develops when the lymphatic system's infection-fighting white blood cells (lymphocytes) grow out of control.
- **T cell** – T cells are lymphocytes that defend against infections that invade your body. In rare cases, though, something goes wrong with the T cells—they change from infection-fighting cells to rapidly multiplying cancer cells.

Peripheral T-cell lymphoma is rare and can be difficult to diagnose and treat. Seek out a medical center that specializes in the diagnosis and treatment of lymphomas.

- **Peripheral** – For T-cell lymphoma, *peripheral* means a cancer that can develop almost anywhere in the body. (So it's unlike a cancer that occurs in a single organ or area, such as the lung or the breast.) Lymphoma can develop almost anywhere in the body because it starts in the lymphatic system, and the lymphatic system exists throughout the body.

Now, let's put it all together:

Peripheral T-cell lymphoma is a cancer that develops from infection-fighting cells found throughout the body in the lymphatic system.

There's a lot more to know about this cancer, though. Importantly, it's not just a single type of lymphoma. Peripheral T-cell lymphoma actually represents a group of many different types of lymphomas. Also important: Peripheral T-cell lymphomas usually grow quickly.

We'll explain more about the different types of peripheral T-cell lymphomas in Chapter 2.

Can peripheral T-cell lymphoma be cured?

Peripheral T-cell lymphomas can be treated and sometimes they can be cured. After treatment, many people have no signs or symptoms of cancer (remission). For most patients, though, the cancer eventually comes back (relapses) at some point after treatment. A relapse usually requires additional treatment.

In the past, the outlook for people with peripheral T-cell lymphoma wasn't good. Even today, the outlook may be discouraging. Most people diagnosed with peripheral T-cell lymphoma will have a difficult road ahead.

But even so, there's hope. Things are changing. New medicines are showing greater effectiveness in treating certain subtypes of peripheral T-cell lymphoma. Also, other promising treatments that are specifically designed to treat peripheral T-cell lymphoma are currently being studied in clinical trials. The number of these trials has increased in recent years, offering more hope for patients.

What is cancer?

Cancer is a disease where cells—the building blocks of the body—grow out of control. This can end up harming the body. There are many types of cells in the body, so there are many types of cancers.

Cancer cells don't behave like normal cells. Normal cells have certain rules. Cancer cells don't follow these rules.

- Cancer cells develop genetic errors (mutations) that allow them to multiply and make many more cancer cells. The cancer cells crowd out and overpower normal cells. Cancer cells take away energy and nutrients that normal cells need.
- Normal cells live for a while and then die. Cancer cells avoid normal cell death. They survive much longer than normal cells do.
- Cancer cells can spread to other areas of the body. They can replace many normal cells and cause organs to stop working well.
- Treatment may get rid of cancer at first but sometimes the cancer comes back later.
- Cancer can stop responding to treatment that worked before.

Scientists have learned a great deal about cancer. As a result, today's treatments work better than treatments in the past. Also, many people with cancer have more treatment choices now than before.

What causes peripheral T-cell lymphoma?

Researchers aren't exactly sure what causes peripheral T-cell lymphoma. What they do know is that these lymphomas start with an abnormality (mutation) in some T-cell lymphocytes. This mutation causes these abnormal T cells to multiply quickly. Before long, the abnormal cells grow out of control. (Cancer is defined by abnormal cells growing out of control.)

The mutation also keeps the abnormal T cells alive much longer than they should live. Eventually, all of these abnormal lymphocytes fill up parts of the lymphatic system. This can cause swelling in the lymph nodes, spleen, liver, or other organs in the body. These problems are also what cause cancer symptoms.

How is peripheral T-cell lymphoma identified?

Peripheral T-cell lymphoma is often found when a person notices a painless lump or swelling in the neck, armpit, or groin. A lump like this is caused by a swollen lymph node.

Peripheral T-cell lymphoma can also occur in parts of the body that aren't lymph nodes. This is called extranodal disease, which means outside the lymph nodes. These areas include the bone marrow, spleen, liver, lungs, kidneys, gastrointestinal (GI) tract, and skin.

Peripheral T-cell lymphoma may also be discovered by certain symptoms. A symptom is a feeling or problem you have that can indicate a disease or condition.

Typical symptoms of peripheral T-cell lymphoma include:

- Fatigue
- Fever
- Night sweats
- Rash
- Unexplained weight loss

Let your doctor know about any symptoms you have. Your symptoms may be the first step toward a diagnosis. A diagnosis involves using tests to identify an illness.

Diagnosing peripheral T-cell lymphoma can be a long and worrisome experience. Many types of lymphoma have similar symptoms. So several tests are required to determine exactly which type of lymphoma you have.

It's important to find the correct diagnosis to get the right treatment.

What are B symptoms?

These three symptoms often occur in people who have lymphoma. They're called B symptoms. Tell your doctor if you have any of these symptoms.

Fever

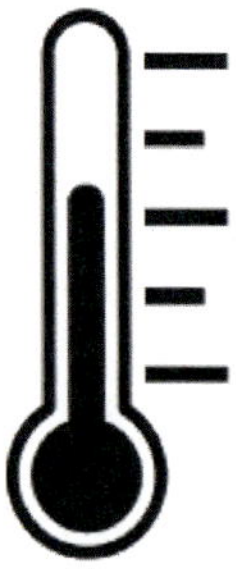

Heavy sweats

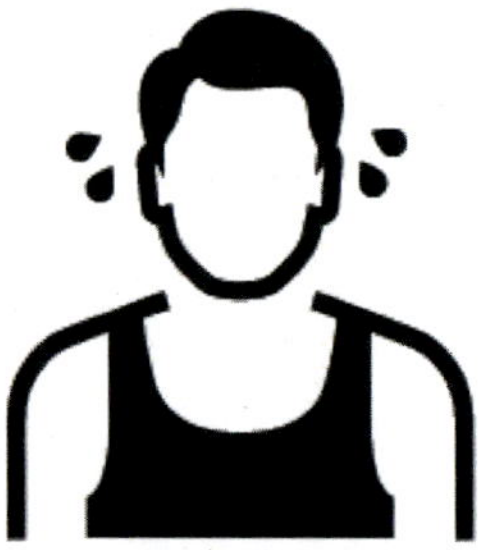

Unexplained weight loss

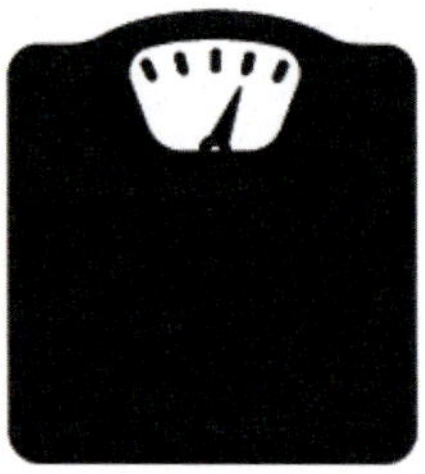

What's the best treatment for peripheral T-cell lymphoma?

There's no single "best" treatment for peripheral T-cell lymphoma. Treatment is focused on you—your age, your current health, how advanced your cancer is, and other factors.

Peripheral T-cell lymphoma is often at an advanced stage when it's diagnosed. But even for advanced lymphomas, treatment is available.

The most common treatment for peripheral T-cell lymphoma is a combination of chemotherapy drugs. Other treatments may include radiation therapy and possibly a bone marrow transplant.

Peripheral T-cell lymphomas can be difficult to treat, so several different types of treatment may be required. Treatment may continue, off and on, for the rest of your life.

It's important to know that cancer treatment today isn't quite as uncomfortable and time-consuming as in the past. A variety of different chemotherapy drugs and treatment options are now available. And there are medications to prevent nausea, vomiting, and other common side effects.

It's also important to know that researchers are constantly studying and developing more effective treatments for cancers like peripheral T-cell lymphoma. Treatments in the future are likely to work better than those that have been available up to now.

Key points

- A lymphoma is a rare cancer that starts in the lymphatic system, which is part of the body's immune system.
- A lymphoma develops when infection-fighting lymphocytes multiply and grow out of control.
- Peripheral T-cell lymphomas are usually fast-growing cancers.
- Peripheral T-cell lymphoma may be discovered when a painless lump is found. Fever, drenching night sweats, and unexplained weight loss may also indicate a lymphoma.
- Diagnosing peripheral T-cell lymphoma can be a long and worrisome experience. You may need many different tests and procedures.
- Peripheral T-cell lymphoma can be difficult to diagnose and treat. Seek out a medical center that specializes in lymphomas.
- It's important to find the correct diagnosis to get the right treatment.
- Peripheral T-cell lymphomas can be treated and sometimes cured.

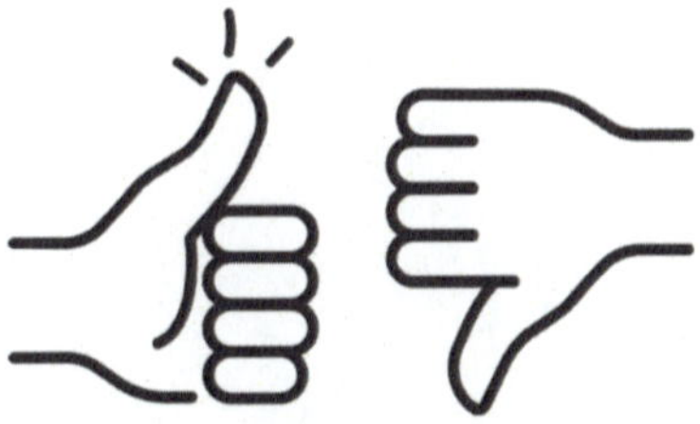

Let us know what you think!

Please take a moment to complete an online survey about the NCCN Guidelines for Patients.

NCCN.org/patients/response

2
Peripheral T-cell lymphoma types

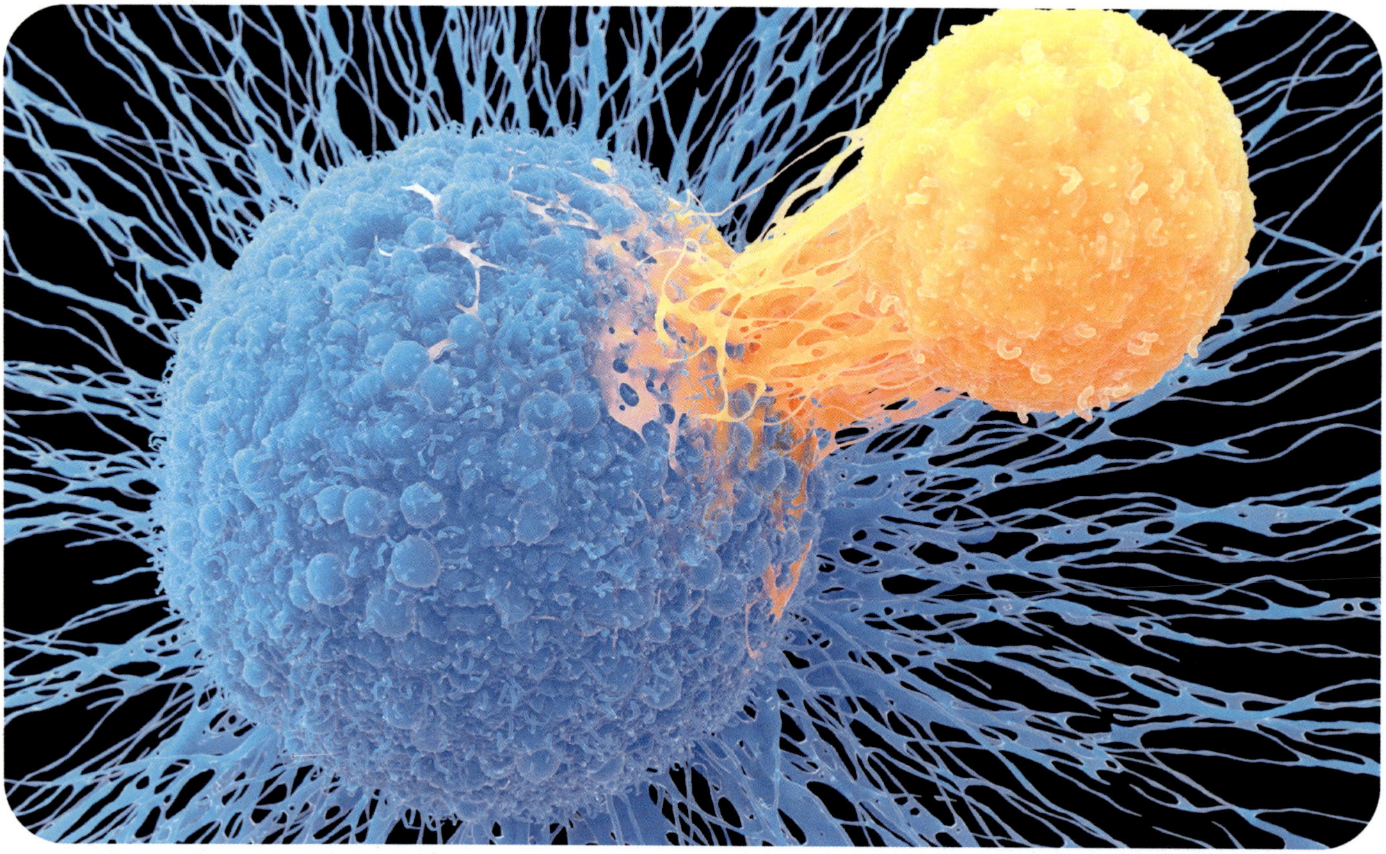

Peripheral T-cell lymphoma is a rare type of cancer. It can be difficult to diagnose, but it's important to try to find out which subtype you have. The more your doctors know about your lymphoma, the more precisely they can treat it.

To understand T-cell lymphomas, we need to understand where they come from and how they grow. T-cell lymphomas, like all lymphomas, develop from lymphocytes (a type of white blood cell) in the lymphatic system.

Lymphatic system

The lymphatic system is part of the immune (infection-fighting) system. The lymphatic system fights germs in the body and transports a fluid called lymph.

The lymphatic system is ma

- lymph fluid
- lymphatic vessels
- lymph nodes
- lymphatic tissue (like bone marrow)
- organs (like the spleen and thymus)

Lymph fluid gives cells water and food. It also contains germ-fighting lymphocytes, including T cells.

As lymph fluid travels through lymphatic vessels throughout the body, lymph nodes catch and filter out foreign particles and harmful cells. Lymph nodes are small, bean-shaped structures. Hundreds of lymph nodes are located throughout the body. Lymph nodes are usually clustered in groups in your neck, chest, armpits, groin, pelvis, and along your gut. (The ones in the neck are often called "glands.")

Lymph nodes

Hundreds of small, bean-shaped structures called lymph nodes are located throughout the human body. Groups of lymph nodes are clustered in your neck, armpits, chest, groin, pelvis, and along your gut. Lymph nodes catch and filter out foreign particles and harmful cells.

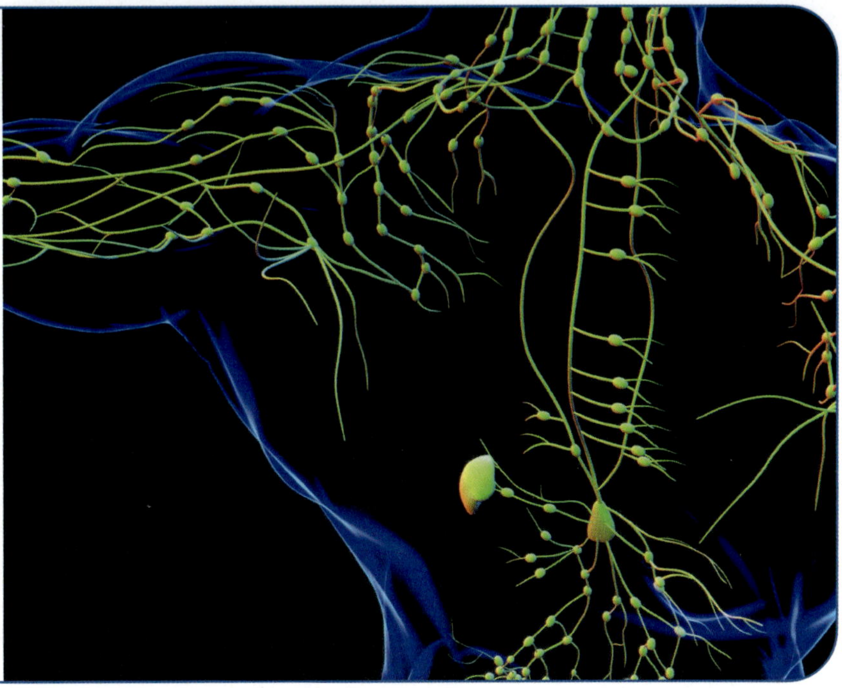

When you get an infection, an army of lymphocytes fills up your lymph nodes to fight the germs. That's why the lymph nodes in your neck feel swollen when you have a cold, the flu, or a sinus infection.

Lymphomas are cancers that start in lymphocytes within the lymphatic system. There are three types of lymphocytes:

- T cells
- B cells
- Natural killer (NK) cells

Like T cells, B cells and NK cells help to fight infections. Lymphomas can develop from these lymphocytes too, namely B-cell lymphomas and NK-cell lymphomas. In this book, we'll focus on T cells.

There are many types of T cells, so there are many T-cell cancers. T cells differ from one another based on the cell's stage of development and what job the T cells have. Very early forms (precursors) of T cells are made in the bone marrow. Bone marrow is a soft, spongy material inside of bones where most blood cells are created.

The immature T cells travel from the bone marrow to the thymus, which is also part of the immune system. In the thymus, the immature T cells develop into mature T cells. (The *T* in thymus gives the T cell its name.) As we get older, immature T cells also develop in

Lymph system

Lymphocytes are produced in bone marrow but further change in lymph tissue to fight disease. The tonsils, thymus, spleen, and lymph nodes are composed of lymph tissue. There are hundreds of lymph nodes in the body and many are in the neck, armpits, and groin.

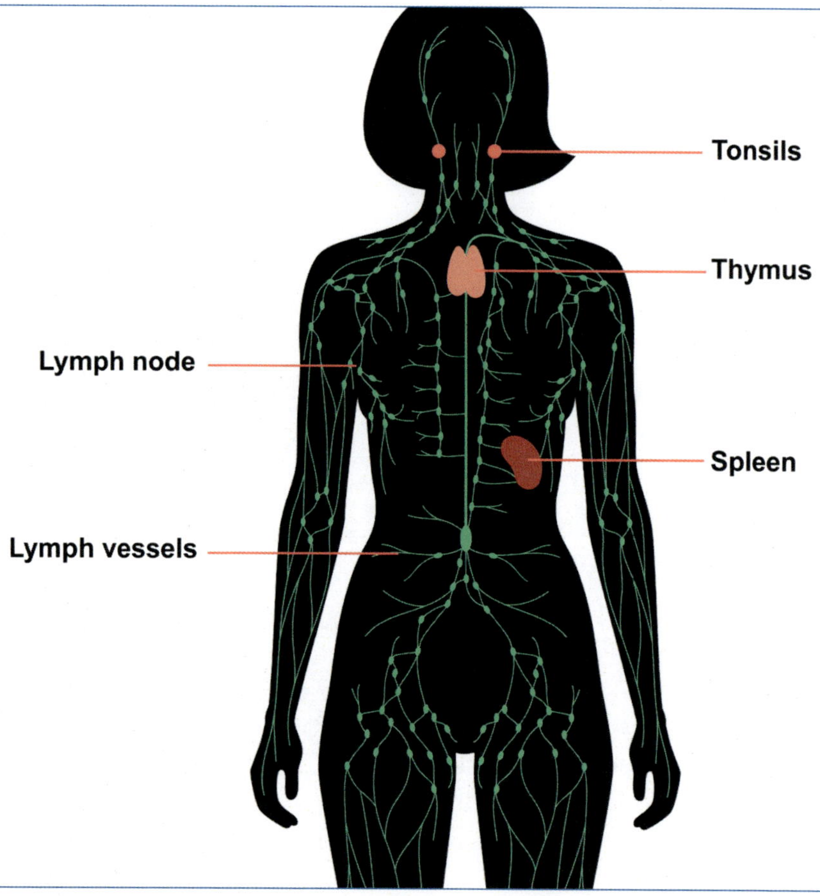

the blood and in other parts of the lymphatic system.

When the T cells are mature, they're ready to help fight illness. They leave the thymus and travel to the lymph nodes and other areas of the lymphatic system. The T cells wait until they're summoned to attack invading germs.

Sometimes these healthy mature T cells can even fight cancer cells. So it's a double loss when T cells develop abnormalities and become cancer cells. Peripheral T-cell lymphoma starts from these abnormal T cells.

Subtypes of peripheral T-cell lymphomas

Peripheral T-cell lymphoma is one of many different types of lymphomas. Lymphomas are divided into two categories: Hodgkin lymphomas and non-Hodgkin lymphomas. Peripheral T-cell lymphoma is a type of non-Hodgkin lymphoma.

Peripheral T-cell lymphoma is a rare disease in the United States. Some forms of peripheral T-cell lymphoma are more common in Asia, Africa, and the Caribbean than in the United States.

Peripheral T-cell lymphoma occurs most often in people aged 60 years and older. But it can also develop in adults younger than 60 and in children. It's diagnosed slightly more often in men than in women.

There are a number of subtypes of peripheral T-cell lymphoma. These subtypes can be very different from one another.

The three most common subtypes are:

Peripheral T-cell lymphoma not otherwise specified (PTCL-NOS)

- Many people with PTCL-NOS have painless swollen lymph nodes in the neck or other parts of the body. In some people, the liver or spleen can be enlarged.
- PTCL-NOS is a diagnosis of exclusion. In other words, a peripheral T-cell lymphoma that doesn't look like any other subtype is categorized as PTCL-NOS.
- PTCL-NOS is also the most common subtype—more than 30% of Americans with peripheral T-cell lymphoma are diagnosed with PTCL-NOS.
- In the United States, PTCL-NOS is more common in Blacks than in Whites.
- PTCL-NOS tends to grow quickly and should be treated as soon as possible.

Angioimmunoblastic T-cell lymphoma (AITL)

- Most people with AITL typically have swollen lymph nodes in the neck or other parts of the body, as well as an enlarged liver or spleen. B symptoms (fevers, night sweats, or unexplained weight loss) are also common.
- AITL is the second most common subtype of peripheral T-cell lymphoma in the United States, accounting for about 15% of all cases.
- In the United States, AITL is more common among Asian/Pacific Islanders and Hispanics than in Whites and Blacks.

- AITL often grows quickly. Treatment usually works in the beginning, but the lymphoma is likely to come back (relapse).

Anaplastic large cell lymphoma (ALCL)

- Most people with ALCL typically have painless swollen lymph nodes in the neck or other parts of the body. B symptoms also often occur.
- This subtype accounts for an estimated 24% of peripheral T-cell lymphoma cases in the United States.
- The ALCL subtype can be either ALK-positive (ALK+) or ALK-negative (ALK−).
- ALK+ ALCL is more common in younger adults while ALK− ALCL is more common in people older than age 55.
- ALK+ ALCL generally has a better prognosis than ALK− ALCL.

In addition to these three most common subtypes of peripheral T-cell lymphoma, many other subtypes also exist. **See Guide 1.**

It's important to try to identify your specific type of T-cell lymphoma to make sure you get the most appropriate care and treatment.

Guide 1. Some common subtypes of peripheral T-cell lymphoma

Subtype	Abbreviation
Peripheral T-cell lymphoma not otherwise specified	PTCL-NOS
Angioimmunoblastic T-cell lymphoma	AITL
Anaplastic lymphoma kinase-positive anaplastic large cell lymphoma	ALK+ ALCL
Anaplastic lymphoma kinase-negative anaplastic large cell lymphoma	ALK− ALCL
Hepatosplenic T-cell lymphoma	HSTCL
Subcutaneous panniculitis-like T-cell lymphoma	SPTCL
Enteropathy-associated T-cell lymphoma	EATL
Monomorphic epitheliotropic intestinal T-cell lymphoma	MEITL
Nodal peripheral T-cell lymphoma with TFH phenotype	Nodal PTCL, TFH
Follicular T-cell lymphoma	FTCL

Key points

- Peripheral T-cell lymphoma starts from T cells that have developed a genetic abnormality.
- Peripheral T-cell lymphoma occurs most often in older adults. But it can also develop in younger adults and children.
- To make sure you get the most appropriate care and treatment, it's important to identify your specific type of T-cell lymphoma.
- There are many subtypes of peripheral T-cell lymphoma. The three most common subtypes in the United States are:
  - Peripheral T-cell lymphoma not otherwise specified (PTCL-NOS)
  - Angioimmunoblastic T-cell lymphoma (AITL)
  - Anaplastic large cell lymphoma (ALCL)

Diagnosis vs. prognosis

What's the difference between your diagnosis and your prognosis? These two words sound alike but they're very different.

Diagnosis means identifying an illness based on tests. Your diagnosis names what illness you have.

Prognosis is the likely course and outcome of a disease based on tests and your response to treatment. Your prognosis predicts how your illness will turn out.

When T cells attack

A healthy T cell (*orange cell*) helps fight infections caused by invaders like bacteria and viruses. Some healthy T cells even fight cancer cells (*blue cell*). So it's a double loss when T cells develop abnormalities and become cancer cells. Peripheral T-cell lymphoma starts from these abnormal T cells.

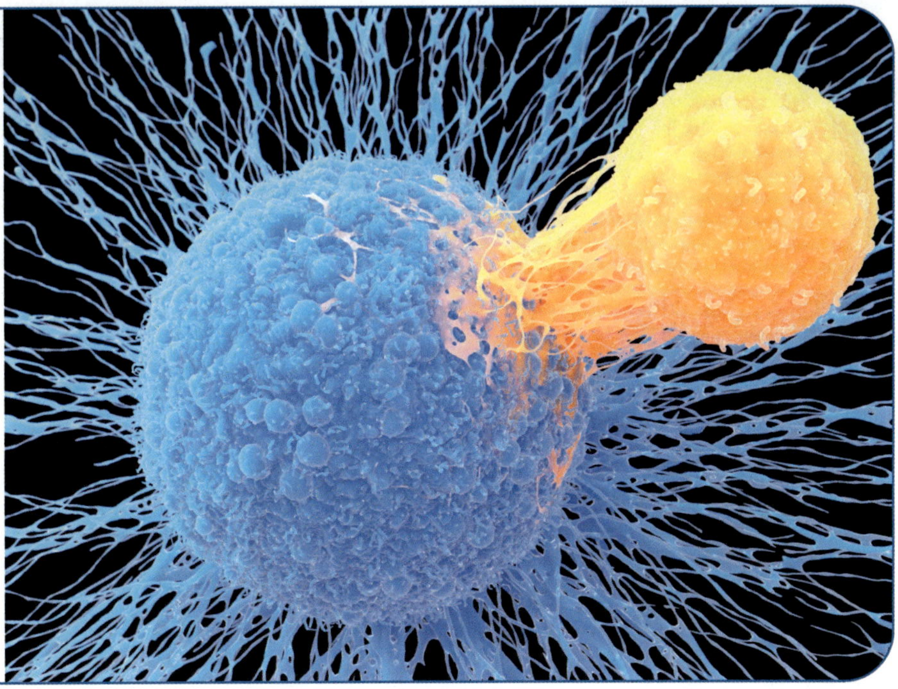

3

Tests you'll take

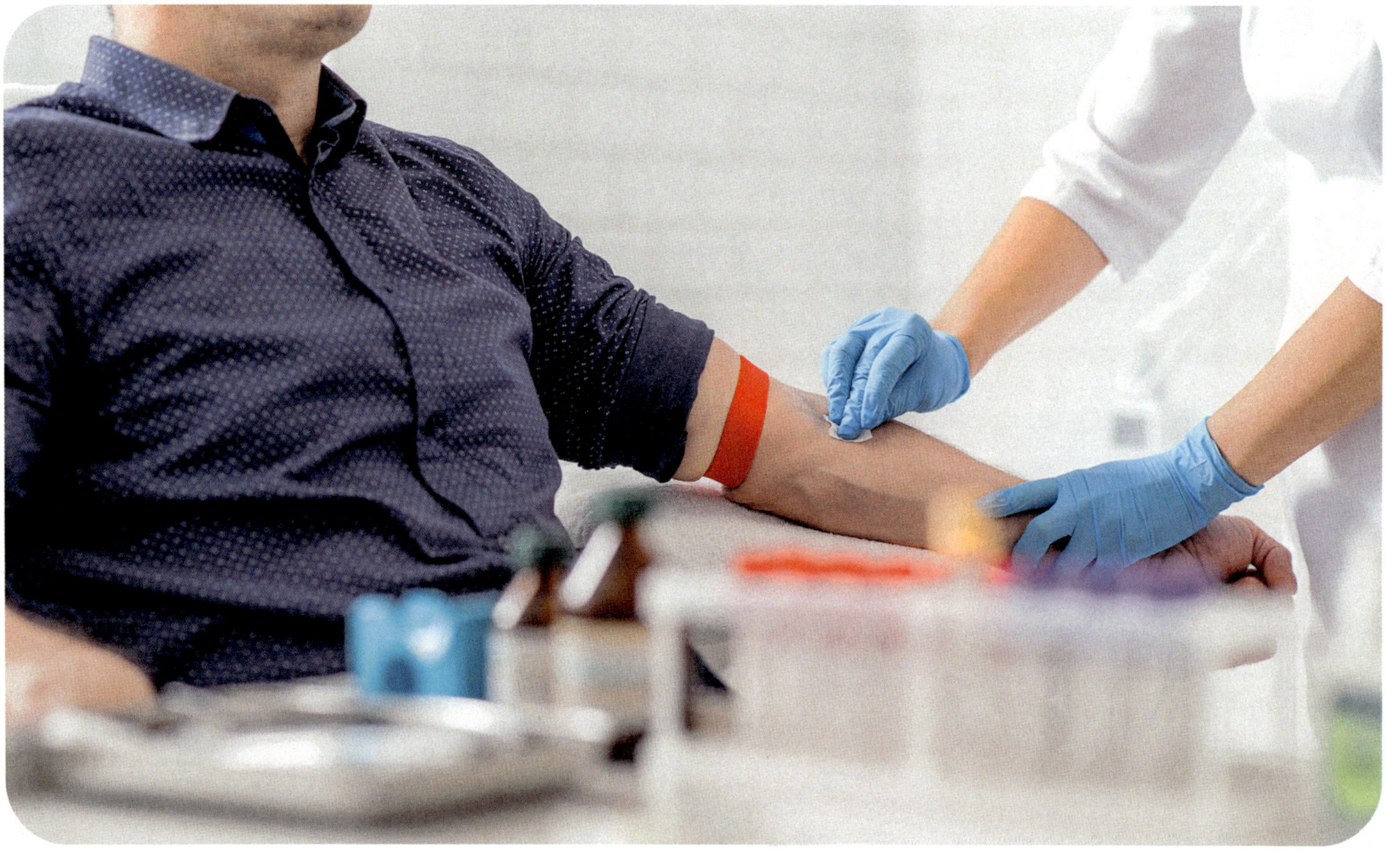

If your doctor suspects that you have peripheral T-cell lymphoma, you'll need a number of medical tests before you receive treatment. Some tests check your general health. Other tests are for diagnosing your illness. All of these tests help to figure out your diagnosis and what treatment is best for you.

The thought of cancer is scary. Having tests for cancer can be scary, too. This chapter will help you know what to expect during testing. Testing will provide a diagnosis, which will help to plan treatment. These steps can help put thoughts into action, which may reduce some of the fear.

It's not easy to find the right diagnosis for peripheral T-cell lymphoma. There's no single test for it. Many different tests are required to make a diagnosis. You'll take some tests more than once, perhaps several times. It's a lot like putting together the pieces of a puzzle to form a picture. Each test adds a new piece to the puzzle.

Of course, not everyone with peripheral T-cell lymphoma may need all the tests described in this chapter.

Tips for testing

Results from blood tests, imaging studies, and biopsies will be used to determine your treatment plan. It's important you understand what these tests mean. Ask questions and keep copies of your test results. Online patient portals are a great way to access your test results.

Remember these tips for testing:

- Bring someone with you to doctor visits, if possible.
- Write down questions and take notes during appointments. Don't be afraid to ask your care team questions. Get to know your care team and let them get to know you.
- Get copies of blood tests, imaging results, and reports about the specific type of cancer you have.
- Organize your papers. Create files for insurance forms, medical records, and test results. You can do the same on your computer.
- Keep a list of contact information for everyone on your care team. Add it to your phone. Hang the list on your refrigerator or keep it in a place where someone can access it in an emergency. Keep your primary care physician informed of changes.

Health history

Your doctors need to have all of your health information. They'll ask you about any health problems and treatments you've had. A complete report of your health is called a medical history.

Medical history, health exams, and other health tests that are used to diagnose peripheral T-cell lymphoma and prepare for treatment are listed in **Guide 2.**

Your doctor will ask about any health problems and treatments you've had during your lifetime. When you meet with your cancer doctors, be ready to talk about:

- Illnesses
- Surgeries
- Injuries
- Health conditions
- Symptoms
- Medications and supplements

Guide 2. Health exams and tests you may need

Health history and exams	• Medical history, including B symptoms • Physical exam, including lymph nodes, liver, spleen, and skin • Performance status
Blood tests	• Complete blood count (CBC) with differential • Comprehensive metabolic panel • Lactate dehydrogenase (LDH) • Uric acid
Infectious disease tests	• Human immunodeficiency virus (HIV) test, if needed • Hepatitis B and C tests, if needed • Human T-cell lymphotropic virus (HTLV) test, if needed
Imaging	• PET/CT scan or CT of chest, abdomen, and pelvis with contrast • CT of neck with contrast, if needed • CT or MRI of head with contrast, if needed
Heart test	• Echocardiogram or MUGA scan, if certain chemotherapy is planned
Biopsies	• Lymph node biopsy • Bone marrow biopsy with or without aspiration • Skin biopsy, if needed • Spinal tap, if needed

Peripheral T-cell lymphoma can cause "B symptoms." Be sure to let your doctor know if you have any of these B symptoms:

- Fevers
- Drenching night sweats
- Unexplained weight loss

Peripheral T-cell lymphoma may also affect other organs, such as your GI tract. (The GI tract is a series of organs—like the stomach and intestines—that break down and digest food.) GI symptoms may include diarrhea, bloody stools, and pain in your belly.

Family history

Some cancers and other health conditions can run in families. T-cell lymphomas typically do not run in families. Be prepared to discuss the health problems of your close blood relatives. These include your brothers and sisters, parents, and grandparents.

Physical exam

A physical exam of your body is done to look for signs of disease. It's also used to help assess what treatments may be options for you. During this exam, your doctor or health care provider may check:

- Your body temperature
- Your blood pressure
- Your pulse and breathing rate
- Your weight
- How your lungs, heart, and gut sound
- How your eyes, skin, nose, ears, and mouth look
- The size of your organs
- Level of pain when you are touched

Swollen glands

Swelling of lymph nodes (such as the "glands" in your throat) is often one of the first signs of lymphoma. Lymph nodes may be so swollen that they can be easily felt or seen under the skin. Your doctor will gently press on the areas of your body that have lymph nodes, such as your neck, armpits, and groin.

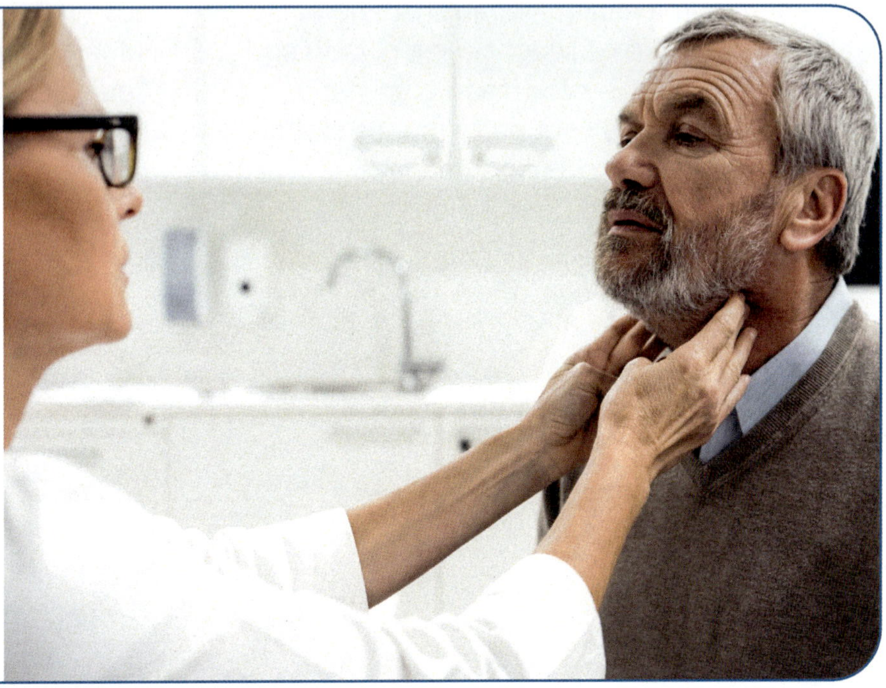

Checking for swelling

Certain parts of your body should be checked for swelling. Swelling of lymph nodes is often one of the first signs of peripheral T-cell lymphoma. Lymph nodes may be so swollen that they can be easily felt or seen under the skin. Your doctor will gently press on the areas of your body that have lymph nodes, such as your neck, armpits, and groin. Your doctor will also feel your spleen and liver to assess their size. Your oropharynx (the back part of your throat, behind your mouth) may also be assessed for signs of cancer, too.

Checking your skin

Another symptom of some peripheral T-cell lymphomas is a rash or rashes on your skin. Your oncologist (a doctor who specializes in cancer) or a dermatologist (a doctor who specializes in skin diseases) may ask to examine the skin on your body.

Checking your physical ability

Your doctor or health care provider will also rate your overall health and ability to do basic daily activities like walking, cleaning, bathing, and so forth. This is known as performance status. Doctors rate your performance status to determine if you can undergo certain treatments. This helps find the treatment that's best suited for you.

Imaging

Imaging makes pictures of the inside of your body. It's used to detect cancer in deep lymph nodes, organs, bone marrow, and other parts of the body. Imaging provides useful information to determine the extent of cancer involvement.

Your treatment team will tell you how to prepare for the test. You may need to stop taking some medicines and stop eating and drinking for a few hours before the scan.

Imaging machines are large. You'll lie down on a table that slides into the machine. At least part of your body will be in the machine. Tell your doctors if you get nervous when in small spaces. You may be given a sedative to help you relax. Imaging machines can also be loud. You'll be given earplugs or headphones to help block out the noise.

After the test, you should be able to resume your normal activities right away. If you took a sedative, you'll be given time to recover. Meanwhile, the scans will be sent to a radiologist for review. A radiologist is a doctor who's an expert in reading the images. The radiologist will send the results of imaging to your doctor.

PET/CT

Positron emission tomography (PET) and computed tomography (CT or CAT scan) are two types of imaging. When used together, they're called a PET/CT scan. The PET/CT scan is used to image your whole body. Some cancer centers have one machine that does both tests at the same time.

- **PET scan** shows whether the cells in your body are functioning normally. It highlights cells that may be cancerous. It can show even small amounts of cancer. A PET scan requires injecting a substance called a radiotracer into your bloodstream. The radiotracer is detected with a special camera during the scan. It makes cancer cells appear brighter on the images. Afterward, the radiotracer is passed out of your body in your urine.
- **CT scan** uses x-rays to take many images of your body from different angles. A computer then combines the pictures to make a 3-D image. If a PET scan isn't available, a CT scan of your chest, belly area, and between your hip bones is needed. A contrast agent (also called contrast dye) is used to make the pictures clearer. Contrast is often injected into the bloodstream and flushed out in urine.

In addition, you may need a CT or magnetic resonance imaging (MRI) scan of your head and a CT scan of your neck to look for cancerous lymph nodes.

PET/CT scan

Imaging instruments, like this PET/CT scanner, can show what's going on inside your body. During the scan, you lie on a table that moves into the tunnel of the machine. The scan can detect even small amounts of cancer.

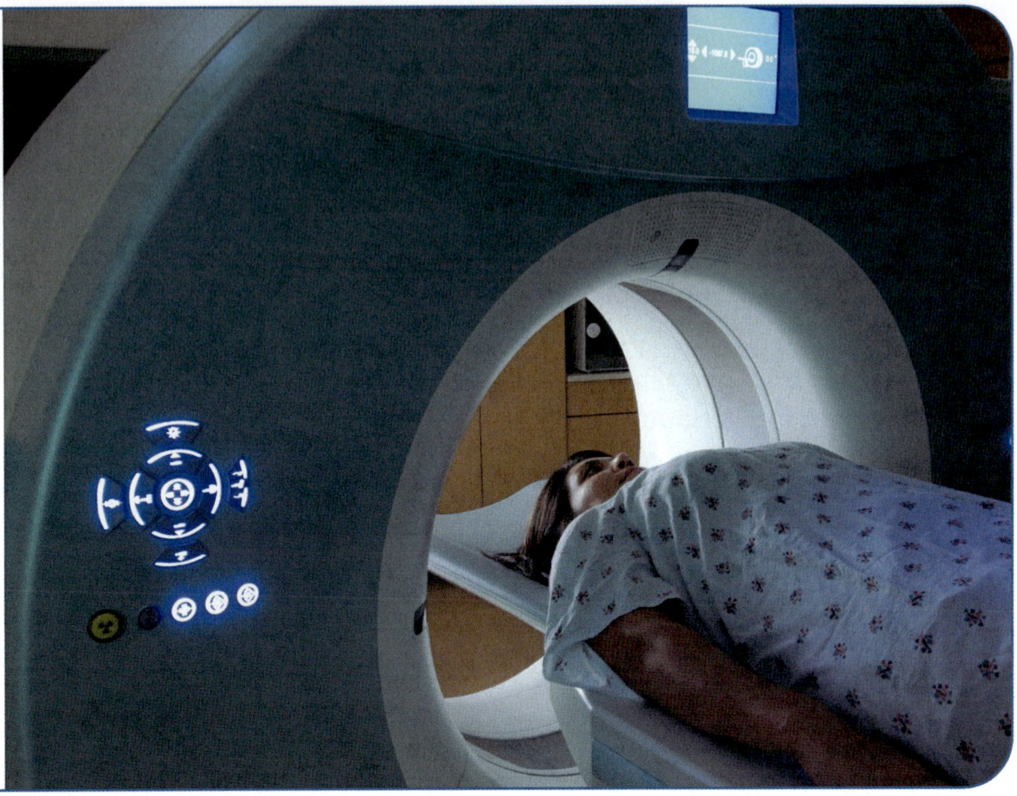

Blood tests

Peripheral T-cell lymphoma can cause abnormal blood counts. Doctors test blood to look for this and other signs of disease. Blood tests are also used to learn when treatment should begin. A sample of your blood is removed with a needle inserted into a vein. This is called a blood draw.

Tests that may be done with your blood sample include:

CBC with differential

A complete blood count (CBC) measures parts of the blood. Test results include measurements of white blood cells, red blood cells, and platelets. Cancer and other health problems can cause low or high counts.

There are five types of white blood cells. A "differential" counts the number of each type of white blood cell. It also checks if the cell counts are in balance with each other. White cell counts that are unusually high or low can suggest the possibility of cancer or other illnesses.

Comprehensive metabolic panel

Your liver, bone, and other organs release chemicals into your blood. A comprehensive metabolic panel includes tests for up to 14 of these chemicals. The tests show if the levels of chemicals are too low or high. Abnormal levels can be caused by cancer or other health problems.

Checking your skin

A rash can be a symptom of peripheral T-cell lymphoma. A doctor may use a dermascope to look at your skin.

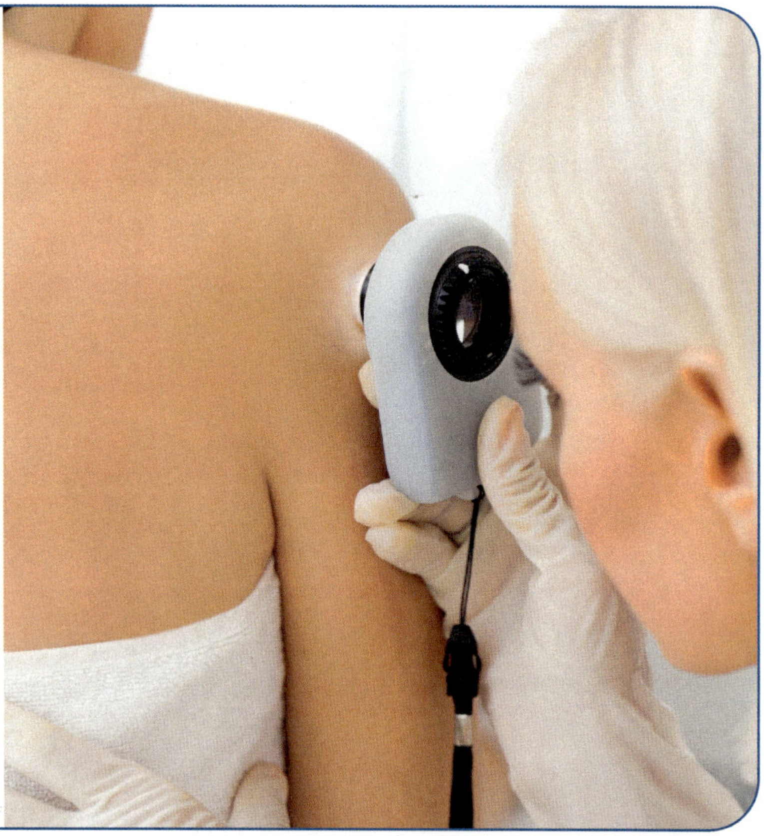

LDH

Lactate dehydrogenase (LDH) is a protein that's in almost all cells. Dying cells release LDH into the blood. High levels of LDH can be caused by cancer or other health problems. If related to lymphoma, high levels may be a sign that treatment may be needed soon.

Uric acid

Uric acid is a normal waste product that's released by cells and is filtered by the kidneys. But high levels of uric acid can be due to fast-growing cancer, kidney disease, or other health problems. High uric acid can also be a side effect of chemotherapy or radiation therapy.

Hepatitis test

Some types of cancer treatments can weaken your immune system. This increases your chance of getting infections. Hepatitis B and hepatitis C infections in particular can become active again after certain cancer therapies. So it's important to be tested for hepatitis viruses before you start treatment.

HIV test

People with human immunodeficiency virus (HIV) tend to have a weakened immune system. So if you have peripheral T-cell lymphoma, it's important to know whether you also have HIV. An HIV antibody test checks for HIV antibodies in a sample of blood, urine, or saliva.

If you haven't been tested for HIV, you may be tested as part of your treatment plan. If you have HIV, treating it is an important part of treating peripheral T-cell lymphoma. Also, cancer treatment works better in people who get treated for their HIV.

Your pathology report

Lab results used for diagnosis are put into a pathology report. This report will be sent to your doctor. It's used to plan your treatment. A meeting among all your doctors may be helpful for treatment planning once the pathology report is finished.

HTLV test

Testing for human T-cell lymphotropic virus (HTLV) can sometimes be helpful for people who appear to have peripheral T-cell lymphoma. In rare cases, HTLV can cause adult T-cell leukemia/lymphoma. This type of T-cell lymphoma can look very similar to peripheral T-cell lymphoma, but is treated differently. So it can be useful to get tested for HTLV to make sure you're being treated for your correct cancer subtype.

Biopsies

The only way to be sure that you have cancer is to test fluid or tissue from your body. A biopsy is a procedure that removes a sample of fluid or tissue for testing. A biopsy is generally a safe test and can often be done in about 30 to 60 minutes.

Several types of biopsies are used to diagnose peripheral T-cell lymphoma:

Lymph node biopsy

Because peripheral T-cell lymphoma typically affects lymph nodes, a lymph node biopsy is common. This biopsy removes lymph node tissue through a cut into your skin.

The duration and complexity of this biopsy depend on the location of the lymph node. If the lymph node is just below the skin, you'll be given a local anesthetic, which numbs only the area of skin and just below the skin. If the lymph node is deeper in the body, you may be given a general anesthetic, which means you'll be asleep during the biopsy.

- An **incisional biopsy** removes only a part of the tissue that may have cancer.
- An **excisional biopsy** removes all of the tissue, such as an entire lymph node.

For either procedure, the surgeon will start by cleaning the skin where the biopsy will be done. Then the surgeon will make a small cut just big enough to remove the lymph node tissue. Lastly, the surgeon will close up the cut with stitches and cover it with a bandage. The tissue sample will be sent to a laboratory after the biopsy is done.

Bone marrow biopsy

Doctors use a bone marrow biopsy and aspiration to remove samples of solid bone marrow and liquid bone marrow for testing. These tests are often done at the same time on the pelvic bone.

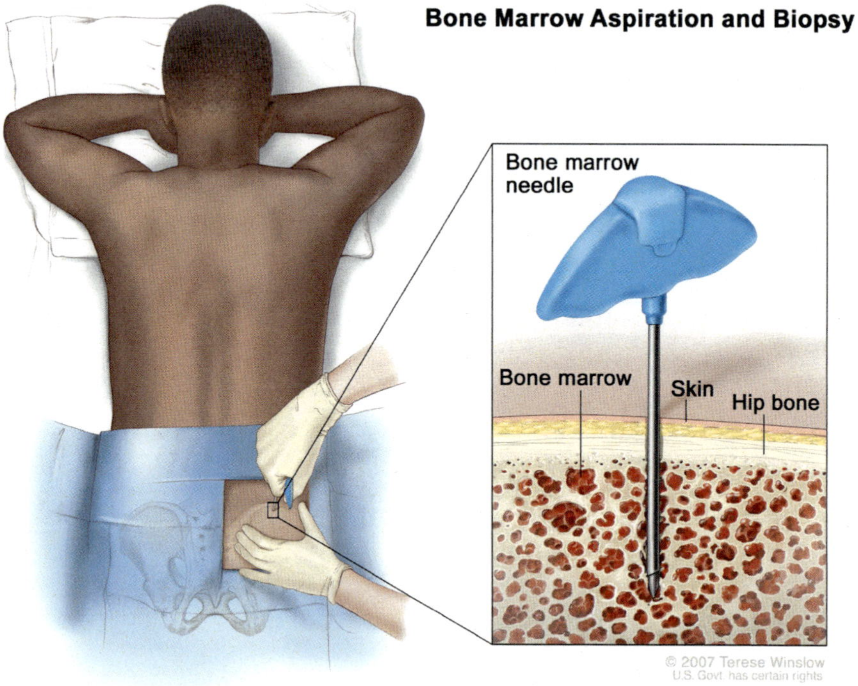

In certain cases when the lymph node is difficult to reach, a core needle biopsy may be done. For a core needle biopsy, the doctor uses a long, hollow needle to remove a small tissue sample (core) from the lymph node.

A biopsy may also be taken from an organ or tissue such as the liver or intestine.

Bone marrow biopsy and aspiration

Peripheral T-cell lymphoma sometimes develops in bone marrow, which is part of the lymph system. You may need a bone marrow biopsy to confirm if there's cancer.

A bone marrow biopsy removes a sample of bone and soft bone marrow. A bone marrow aspiration removes liquid bone marrow. Both procedures are often done at the same time on the back of the hip bone, which contains a large amount of bone marrow.

You may receive a light sedative before the test to help you relax. Your doctor will then clean the area and you'll be given anesthesia to numb the skin and the bone beneath.

Once the area is numb, a hollow needle will be inserted into the bone and rotated to remove a sample of bone and soft marrow. You'll notice a feeling of pressure as this is happening and you might feel some pain while the samples are being removed. Afterward, your skin may be bruised for a few days. After the tissue samples are collected, they'll be sent to a lab for testing.

Skin biopsy

Peripheral T-cell lymphomas and other T-cell lymphomas may involve the skin. Based on your skin exam, your doctor may want you to have a skin biopsy. A skin biopsy removes a sample of one or two layers of skin, which is tested for cancer.

Before the biopsy, the area of skin will be numbed with anesthesia. You may feel pressure during the biopsy. Afterward, your doctor will close the wound and apply a bandage. There are usually no side effects, but some people do get scars.

Diagnostic tests

Cancers of blood cells are difficult to tell apart. Diagnostic tests can help reveal which cancer you have.

For these tests, your blood and tissue samples will be sent to a laboratory. At the laboratory, a doctor called a hematopathologist will view the samples under a microscope. Hematopathologists are experts at diagnosing cancers of blood cells. They can identify different types of cancer by viewing the size, shape, and arrangement of cells under the microscope.

If cancer cells are found, the hematopathologist will test the cells for certain proteins and genetic abnormalities. It often takes several days before the test results are known.

Diagnostic tests that may be performed on your samples include protein tests and biomarker tests.

Protein tests

Cancer cells can be detected by specific proteins found on the surface of the cells. The presence or absence of these proteins can help determine the diagnosis and type of the cancer. That is, each subtype of peripheral T-cell lymphoma has its own pattern or "signature" of proteins. This is called immunophenotyping.

By detecting this "signature," the hematopathologist can diagnose a subtype based on which proteins it has and which ones it doesn't have. For example, a specific subtype of peripheral T-cell lymphoma may have the CD4 protein but not the CD5 protein.

Immunophenotyping for peripheral T-cell lymphoma also typically looks for proteins CD2, CD3, CD7, CD8, CD10, CD20, CD30, BCL6, Ki-67, ALK, and many others. Each of these proteins performs a different job for the cell.

Besides identifying the subtype, immunophenotyping is used to estimate how aggressive the cancer is.

Immunophenotyping can also suggest which type of treatment might work best against the cancer. For example, anaplastic large cell lymphoma (ALCL) is a subtype that has a lot of CD30 protein. Scientists have developed a treatment—brentuximab vedotin—that targets and destroys cancer cells with the CD30 protein. So the preferred treatment for the ALCL subtype now includes brentuximab vedotin. Newer treatments like this are often more effective and may have fewer side effects than standard chemotherapy.

Biomarker tests

Biomarker testing looks for biological clues of cancer. Biomarkers can be genes, proteins, or genetic changes (mutations). They can be found in your tissues, blood, or other bodily fluids.

Biomarker testing can be used to:

- Confirm or support the diagnosis of a person's cancer
- Tell the difference between one cancer type and another
- Clarify the prognosis of a person's cancer
- Help choose the most appropriate treatment

Doctors can use biomarkers to help identify some peripheral T-cell lymphoma subtypes and choose the right treatment for them. For example, certain genetic abnormalities can point to specific subtypes, such as ALK+ ALCL. In this subtype, a specific genetic abnormality—a rearrangement of the anaplastic lymphoma kinase (*ALK*) gene—is found in all cases of ALK+ ALCL.

But there is much more to learn. Scientists are constantly looking for more biomarkers that can provide more answers for better diagnosis and treatment of peripheral T-cell lymphoma.

Ask if the hematopathologist who's testing your samples has experience in diagnosing peripheral T-cell lymphoma.

Fertility and pregnancy

Some cancer treatments may affect your ability to conceive or bear children. However, options are available. Sperm can be frozen and stored in a sperm bank until after cancer treatment. Like sperm banking, eggs can be removed from ovaries and stored for later use. Discuss your thoughts and preferences with your doctors.

Some cancer treatments can harm an unborn baby. If you might be pregnant now, get a pregnancy test before your treatment. Also, take steps to avoid getting pregnant or causing a pregnancy during treatment. Your doctors can tell you which birth control methods are best to use.

Heart tests

Some cancer treatments can damage your heart. To plan treatment, your doctor may test how well your heart is working. You may get an echocardiogram or a multigated acquisition (MUGA) scan. An echocardiogram uses sound waves to make pictures of your heart. A MUGA scan makes pictures using a radiotracer and a special camera. If your heart isn't working well, your doctor may avoid using certain chemotherapy drugs that could cause further damage to your heart.

Staging

Staging is a method that oncologists use to describe the extent of cancer in the body. It's based on the results of a person's imaging scans, biopsies, and blood tests. Staging can be used to estimate your prognosis and to help choose the best treatment or the right clinical trial for you.

Staging is often described as early stage or late (advanced) stage. This is expressed using numbers 1 to 4. Early stage disease is defined as stage 1 and 2 while late or advanced stage disease is stage 3 and 4. For peripheral T-cell lymphoma, the cancer stages are:

- **Stage 1** – Cancer in one lymph node or a single cluster of lymph nodes
- **Stage 2** – Cancer in two or more groups of lymph nodes in the same area of the body
- **Stage 3** – Cancer in lymph nodes in different areas of the body or cancer in lymph nodes in the same area of the body and in the spleen
- **Stage 4** – Stage 1, 2, or 3 plus cancer found in other organs like the liver, lung, kidneys, GI tract, or bone marrow

Staging is helpful to make treatment decisions. It helps determine if you need systemic treatment alone or if systemic treatment should be combined with local treatment like radiation. Systemic treatment affects the entire body.

To read more about your initial treatment options, turn to Chapter 4.

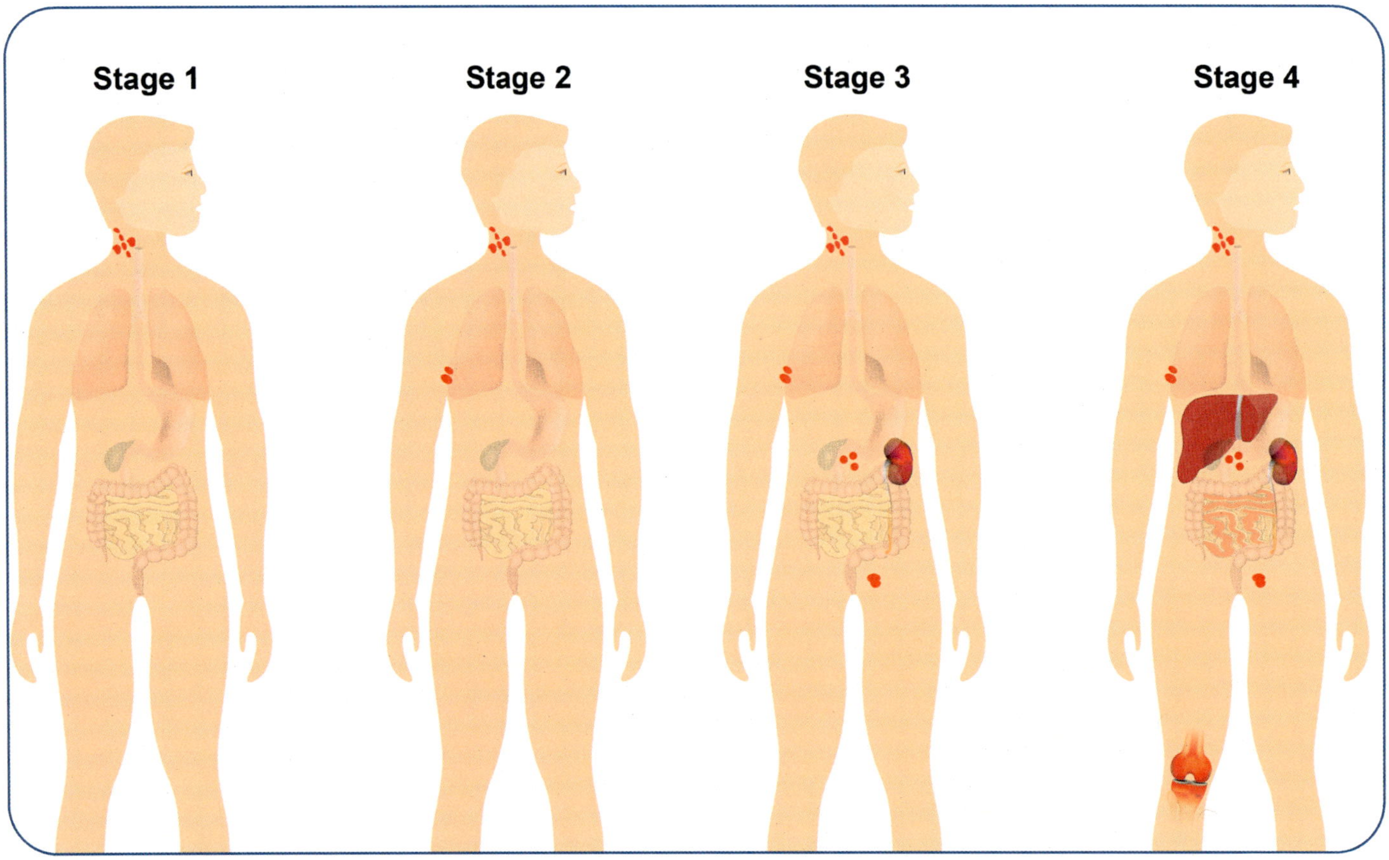

Key points

- There's no single test for peripheral T-cell lymphoma. Many different tests are required to make a diagnosis.
- Your doctor will ask about any health problems and treatments you've had in your lifetime.
- Tell your doctor if you have recently had fevers, night sweats, or weight loss. These can be symptoms of lymphoma.
- Your doctor will check the areas of your body that have lymph nodes. Swelling of lymph nodes is often one of the first signs of peripheral T-cell lymphoma.
- Blood tests look for signs of cancer and other health problems.
- Imaging tests allow your doctors to see inside your body without cutting into it. Imaging scans show the amount of cancer and where the cancer is located.
- An incisional or excisional biopsy is the only sure way to diagnose cancer. Other types of biopsy may also be needed.
- Protein tests identify a signature-like pattern of proteins that can reveal whether you have peripheral T-cell or another type of lymphoma.
- Molecular tests and DNA sequencing can find genetic abnormalities and mutations that may provide both the diagnosis and prognosis of cancer.
- Your doctor will use the results of all these tests to assess the outlook (prognosis) of your cancer.
- Some cancer treatments can harm an unborn baby. If you might be pregnant, get a pregnancy test before treatment.

4 First-line therapy

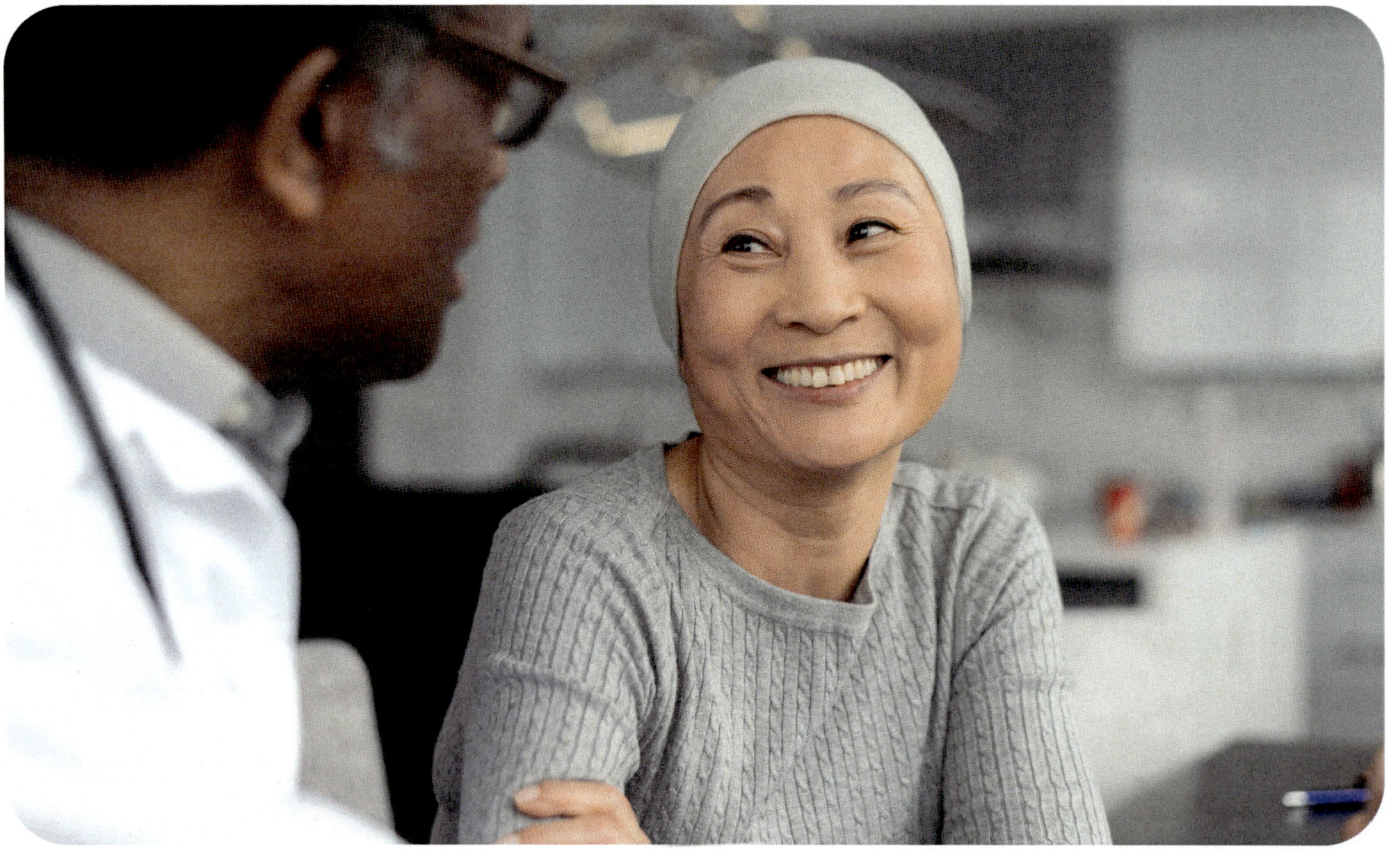

There's no single best treatment for peripheral T-cell lymphoma—there are a number of options for different people. The first and most promising type of treatment is called first-line therapy.

There are many ways to try to treat a peripheral T-cell lymphoma, but none is perfect. So your treatment team will gather all the details about your lymphoma and your health to choose the right treatments for you. Treatments are based on:

- The stage of lymphoma
- The size and location of the lymphoma
- How the lymphoma is affecting your body
- Your symptoms
- Your age
- Your medical history
- Your physical and mental condition
- Your preferences and concerns

Your treatment team will look at all these things to come up with the best possible treatment plan. The plan will likely include several types of treatment over time. This plan will involve a range of health care providers. The beginning treatment is called first-line therapy.

What is first-line therapy?

First-line therapy (also known as upfront treatment) is the first type of treatment given for a condition or disease. A first-line treatment is one that generally provides the best results with the fewest side effects. A side effect is an unhealthy or unpleasant physical or emotional condition caused by treatment.

The goal of first-line therapy is to be cured, if possible. If a cure is not possible, then the goal is to achieve long-term remission or control of the cancer. Remission means the cancer isn't detectable and isn't causing any symptoms after treatment.

First-line therapy can be a single type of treatment, such as chemotherapy, or it can be a combination of treatments, such as chemotherapy and radiation therapy. Sometimes two or more treatments are used together for a greater effect.

First-line therapy

. . . is the first treatment program given for a disease. First-line therapy is the one considered to be the best treatment.

Second-line therapy

. . . is the next treatment given if first-line therapy isn't working or stops working.

For peripheral T-cell lymphoma, three first-line treatment options are available:

- Chemotherapy
- Radiation therapy
- Clinical trial

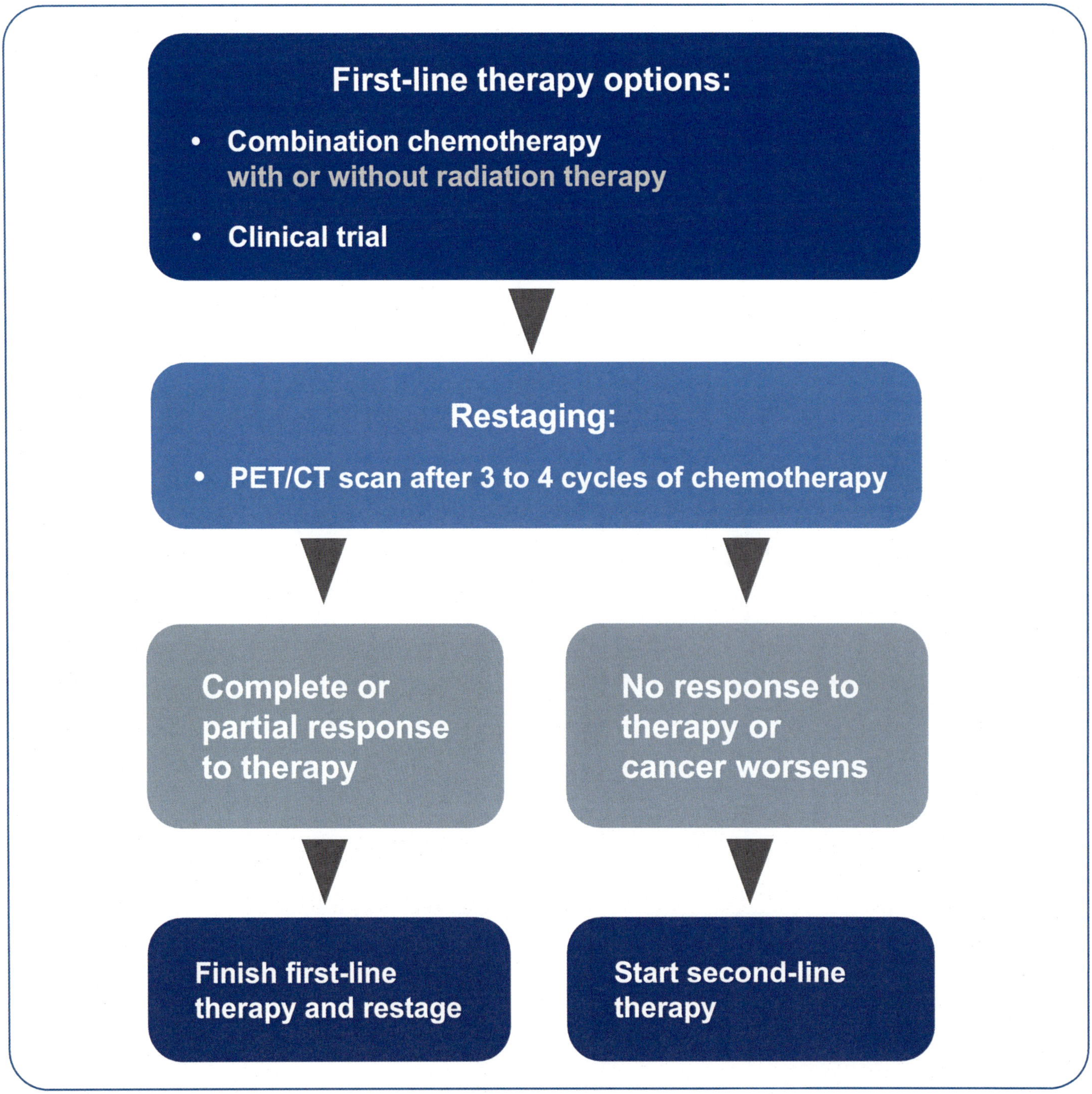

Chemotherapy

Chemotherapy ("chemo") is the use of drugs to kill cancer cells. Chemotherapy drugs kill fast-growing cells throughout the body. Cancer cells are fast-growing cells, but some normal cells are fast-growing, too. Different types of chemotherapy drugs work in different ways to kill cancer cells or stop new ones from being made.

Many chemotherapy drugs are liquids that are injected slowly into a vein (IV infusion). Some are pills that are swallowed. The drugs travel in the bloodstream to treat cancer throughout the body. Treatment that affects the whole body is called systemic therapy.

For peripheral T-cell lymphoma treatment, a few chemotherapy drugs are often given at the same time. This is called multi-agent or combination chemotherapy. The advantage of multi-agent chemotherapy is that each drug has its own way of attacking the lymphoma. This gives the combination a better chance of overpowering the cancer. Plus, it's much harder for the cancer to develop resistance to a combination of drugs than to a single drug. **See Guide 3.**

Guide 3. Recommended first-line chemotherapy combinations for treating peripheral T-cell lymphoma

Chemotherapy combination	Abbreviation
• brentuximab vedotin • cyclophosphamide • doxorubicin • prednisone	BVCHP
• cyclophosphamide • doxorubicin • vincristine • prednisone	CHOP
• cyclophosphamide • doxorubicin • vincristine • etoposide • prednisone	CHOEP
• etoposide • prednisone • vincristine • cyclophosphamide • doxorubicin	EPOCH

These regimens are listed in alphabetical order, not in order of importance.

Medicines used in first-line chemotherapy combinations

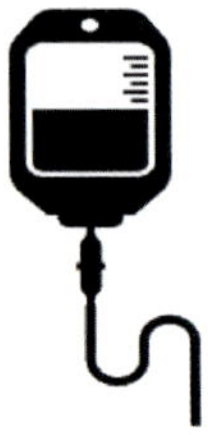

Certain medicines that aren't chemotherapeutic drugs are often given as part of first-line chemotherapy combinations. For example, one of the preferred first-line therapy regimens for peripheral T-cell lymphoma consists of a drug conjugate (brentuximab vedotin), two chemotherapy drugs (cyclophosphamide and doxorubicin), and a corticosteroid (prednisone). These drugs can boost the overall effect of chemotherapy and may help reduce side effects.

Brentuximab vedotin

- Brentuximab vedotin is a drug conjugate used as a first-line treatment for peripheral T-cell lymphomas that have the CD30 protein. A drug conjugate combines two drugs in one medicine: One drug finds and binds to certain cancer cells and the other drug directly attacks the cancer cells without harming other cells. Brentuximab vedotin is called a targeted therapy because it specifically targets cancer cells that have the CD30 protein.
- *The most common side effects of brentuximab vedotin include fatigue, low blood counts, tingling or numbness in hands and feet, nausea, diarrhea, fever, rash, and lung infections. Rare but severe side effects include brain infection, serious disorder of skin and mucous membranes, and kidney problems.*

Corticosteroids (often called "steroids")

- These drugs are used to relieve swelling and inflammation. Some steroids also have anti-cancer effects. Plus, steroids help chemotherapy to work better and reduce side effects like fatigue, nausea, and loss of appetite. Steroids may be given as a pill, a liquid, or an IV injection.
- *Common side effects of steroids include feeling hungry, trouble sleeping, mood changes, slow wound healing, upset stomach, and swelling in the ankles, feet, and hands. Side effects usually fade away once the steroid is stopped.*

Growth factors

- Growth factors are drugs that boost the immune system. Chemotherapy can weaken the immune system. Growth factors help restore your immune system after chemotherapy. Growth factors can be given as a daily injection under the skin or as a single injection that keeps working in the body for several weeks. Not everyone who receives chemotherapy needs growth factors.

Treatment for peripheral T-cell lymphoma usually involves a mix of liquid drugs. You'll sit in a chair or bed at the hospital or clinic while receiving the medicine. A treatment session can range from a few minutes to a few hours.

Chemotherapy is given in cycles of treatment days followed by days of rest. This allows the body to recover before the next treatment cycle. Cycles vary in length depending on which drugs are used. Often, the cycles are 14, 21, or 28 days long. The number of treatment days per cycle and the total number of cycles given also vary based on the chemotherapy used.

Common side effects of chemotherapy are nausea, vomiting, diarrhea, mouth sores, loss of appetite, hair loss, and low blood cell counts. Feeling very tired (fatigue) or weak is also common.

Don't disregard a fever

Chemotherapy can weaken your immune system and make you more likely to get infections. One sign of an infection is a fever. If you have a fever while receiving chemotherapy, you need to contact your treatment team. Make sure to ask for a phone number you can call if you get a fever or have another urgent problem.

What is chemotherapy?

Chemotherapy ("chemo") is the use of drugs to kill cancer cells. The drug is often a liquid medicine that's infused (slowly injected) into your arm while you sit in a chair. Some people, like this man, receive chemo through a port implanted in their chest.

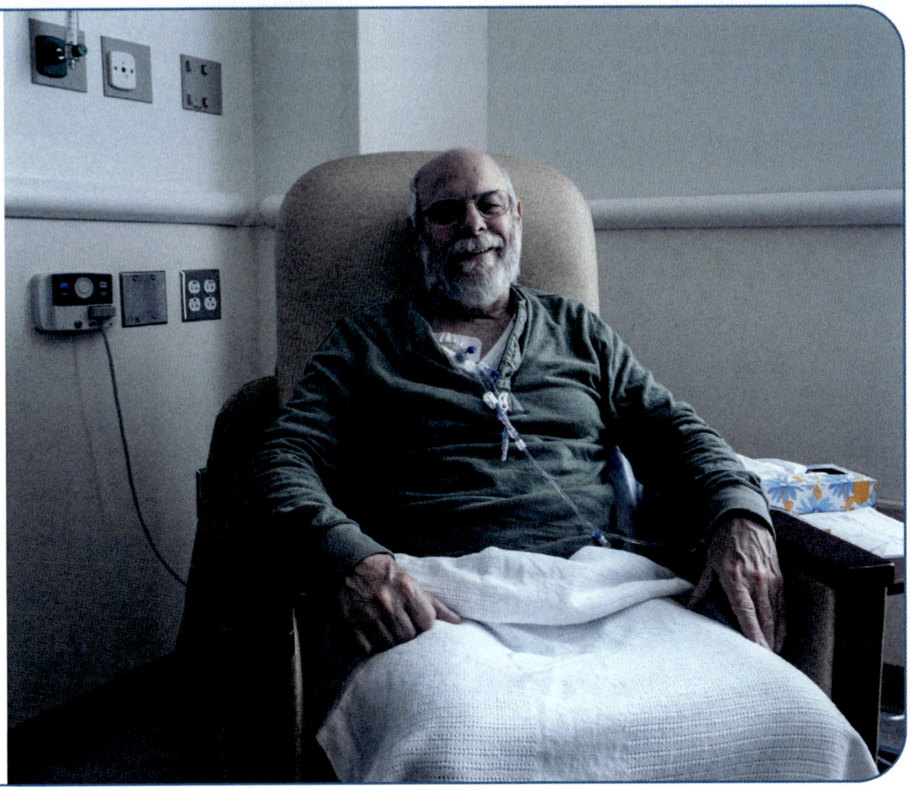

Side effects of chemotherapy are generally caused by the death of fast-growing cells, which are found in the intestines, mouth, blood, skin, and hair follicles. But the side effects of chemotherapy depend on many other factors, too. These include the drug, the dose, and the person.

Not everyone experiences the same side effects or number of side effects. Also, not all side effects of chemotherapy are listed here. Ask your treatment team for a complete list of common and rare side effects. If any side effect bothers you, tell your treatment team. There may be ways to help you feel better. There are also ways to prevent some side effects.

Radiation therapy

For peripheral T-cell lymphoma, radiation therapy is given in very specific instances after chemotherapy as part of first-line treatment. Radiation therapy is used to destroy any remaining cancer cells that are left behind after chemo.

In people who can't have chemotherapy, radiation therapy may be used alone to relieve pain or other symptoms caused by the lymphoma or by other treatment.

Radiation therapy involves a large machine that sends out high-energy rays to a specific area of the body. The rays damage the DNA in cancer cells. This either kills the cancer cells or stops new cancer cells from being made. You won't see, hear, or feel the radiation. It passes

What is radiation therapy?

Radiation therapy is the use of high-energy radiation to kill cancer cells.

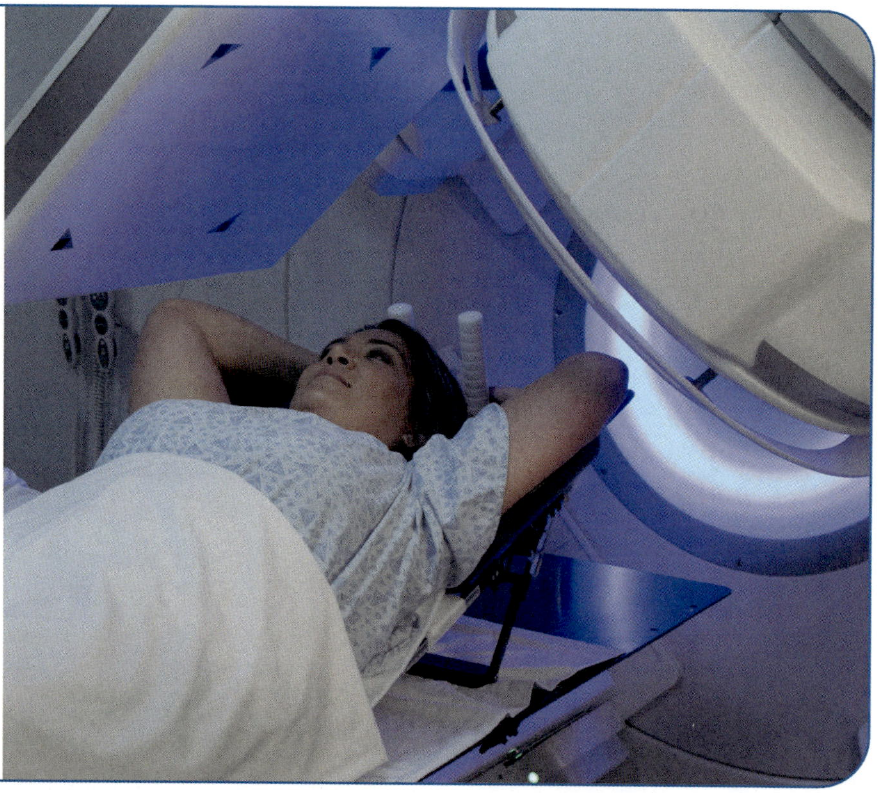

through your skin and other tissues to reach the lymphoma. (Radiation therapy won't make you radioactive.)

Radiation therapy is a type of local therapy. Local therapy treats cancer cells only in a specific area of the body. If you're having radiation therapy, a radiation oncologist will come up with a treatment plan that tries to avoid harming any important organs or other parts of your body. To help accomplish this, imaging with CT, PET, or MRI may be needed to plan or to perform radiation therapy.

During treatment, you'll lie on the treatment table and be told how to get into position needed for treatment. You need to remain very still during radiation treatment. Devices may be used to keep you from moving.

You'll be alone in the room while the radiology technician operates the machine from a nearby control room. The technician will be able to see, hear, and speak with you through an intercom and video system. One treatment session takes about 15 to 30 minutes—only a few minutes of the session involve actual radiation time. Radiation therapy usually requires a series of treatment sessions over several weeks.

Side effects of radiation therapy differ among people. Factors like the location of the radiation on your body, radiation dose, and length of treatment all play a role. Side effects are cumulative, meaning they may not be too severe in the first few visits but will get worse over the course of treatment. Over time, you may have nausea, diarrhea, or fatigue. You may lose your appetite and may even lose weight during treatment.

Other side effects occur in treated areas, such as redness of the skin or hair loss. The side effects of radiation therapy usually go away by 2 to 4 weeks after the treatment ends.

Clinical trial

A clinical trial is a type of medical research study. After being developed and tested in a laboratory, potential new ways of fighting cancer need to be studied in people. If found to be safe and effective in a clinical trial, a drug, device, or treatment approach may be approved by the U.S. Food and Drug Administration (FDA).

Participating in a clinical trial isn't a "last-ditch" effort. A clinical trial is a first-line treatment option for many people with lymphoma. Clinical trials give people access to options that they couldn't usually receive otherwise. Everyone with cancer should carefully consider all of the treatment options available for their cancer type, including standard treatments and clinical trials.

NCCN recommends that people with peripheral T-cell lymphoma consider a clinical trial as their first-line therapy, if available.

Talk to your doctors about whether a clinical trial is recommended for you.

Phases

Most cancer clinical trials focus on treatment. Treatment trials are done in phases.

- **Phase I trials** study the dose, safety, and side effects of a drug or treatment approach. They also look for early signs that the drug or approach is helpful.
- **Phase II trials** study how well the drug or approach works against a specific type of cancer.
- **Phase III trials** test the drug or approach against a standard treatment. If the results are good, it may be approved by the FDA.
- **Phase IV trials** study the long-term safety and benefit of an FDA-approved treatment.

Who can enroll?

Every clinical trial has rules for joining, called eligibility criteria. The rules may be about age, cancer type and stage, treatment history, or general health. These requirements ensure that participants are alike in specific ways and that the trial is as safe as possible for the participants.

Informed consent

Clinical trials are managed by a group of experts called a research team. The research team will review the study with you in detail, including its purpose and the risks and benefits of joining. All of this information is also provided in an informed consent form. Read the form carefully and ask questions before signing it. Take time to discuss with family, friends, or other people who you trust. Keep in mind that you can leave and seek treatment outside of the clinical trial at any time.

Start the conversation

Don't wait for your doctor to bring up clinical trials. Start the conversation and learn about all of your treatment options. If you find a study that you may be eligible for, ask your treatment team if you meet the requirements. If you've already started standard treatment, you may not be eligible for certain clinical trials. Try not to be discouraged if you can't join. New clinical trials are always becoming available.

Frequently asked questions

There are many myths and misconceptions surrounding clinical trials. The possible benefits and risks are not well understood by many with cancer.

› Will I get a placebo?

Placebos (inactive versions of real medicines) are almost never used alone in cancer clinical trials. It's common to receive either a placebo with a standard treatment, or a new drug with a standard treatment. You'll be informed, verbally and in writing, if a placebo is part of a clinical trial before you enroll.

› Are clinical trials free?

There's no fee to enroll in a clinical trial. The study sponsor pays for research-related costs, including the study drug. You may, however, have costs indirectly related to the trial, such as the cost of transportation or child care due to extra appointments. During the trial, you'll continue to receive standard cancer care. This care is billed to—and often covered by—insurance. You're responsible for copays and any costs for this care that aren't covered by your insurance.

Finding a clinical trial

In the United States

NCCN Cancer Centers
NCCN.org/cancercenters

The National Cancer Institute (NCI)
cancer.gov/about-cancer/treatment/clinical-trials/search

Worldwide

The U.S. National Library of Medicine (NLM)
clinicaltrials.gov

Need help finding a clinical trial?

NCI's Cancer Information Service (CIS)
1.800.4.CANCER (1.800.422.6237)
cancer.gov/contact

Restaging

You read about staging in Chapter 3. Restaging means evaluating the extent of a person's cancer after some treatment has been given. Restaging can occur during the middle of treatment to check how well it's working. Restaging can also be done after treatment is over or if the cancer comes back or has spread.

During restaging, you'll repeat some of the same tests that you did before you were first diagnosed. For peripheral T-cell lymphoma, restaging occurs after 3 or 4 cycles of first-line chemotherapy and is done with PET/CT or other imaging. The results give doctors an idea of how your cancer is responding to treatment.

Responses to treatment:

- Complete response means there are no signs of lymphoma after treatment.
- Partial response is when the size or extent of the lymphoma has decreased after treatment.
- No response after treatment means the cancer is stable with no significant change—it didn't grow but it didn't shrink.
- Progressive disease means that the cancer is growing and/or spreading despite treatment.

What's next? It depends on how well the lymphoma responds to treatment:

No response or progressive disease

People who have no response or progressive disease will move on to second-line therapy.

To read about second-line therapy, go to Chapter 5.

Complete response or partial response

People who have a complete response or a partial response to first-line therapy will finish the treatment and be restaged again. They may have additional therapy or something called consolidation therapy. For more information about additional and consolidation therapy, turn to Chapter 6.

Two types of survival

You may hear or read about different terms for survival, such as overall survival and progression-free survival. In a clinical trial, measuring either form of survival can show how well a new treatment works. But what do these terms really mean?

Overall survival: How long a person remains alive after the start of their cancer. The "start of their cancer" can be either the date it's diagnosed or the date when treatment begins.

Progression-free survival: How long a person goes after the start of treatment without the cancer getting worse.

Key points

- Your treatment plan will likely include several types of treatment over time. You'll also meet with a range of health care providers.
- First-line therapy generally provides the best results with the fewest side effects.
- Chemotherapy is the use of drugs to kill cancer cells.
- For peripheral T-cell lymphoma, radiation therapy is used to destroy any remaining cancer cells that are left behind after chemotherapy.
- A clinical trial is a first-line treatment option for many people with lymphoma.
- Clinical trials give people access to treatment options that they couldn't usually receive otherwise.

Restaging means evaluating a person's cancer after treatment has been given.

What is a regimen?

A regimen is a plan that defines the dosage, schedule, and duration of a treatment. Regimens for peripheral T-cell lymphoma often include multiple drugs.

It's normal to feel worried

Depression, anxiety, fear, and distress are very common feelings in people with cancer. These feelings can make it harder to deal with cancer and cancer treatment. They can hold you back even when you want to move forward. Getting help when you're feeling worried or hopeless is an important part of cancer care. If you're feeling anxious or overwhelmed, ask your treatment team for help.

Read more about cancer and distress in *NCCN Guidelines for Patients: Distress During Cancer Care*, available at NCCN.org/patientguidelines.

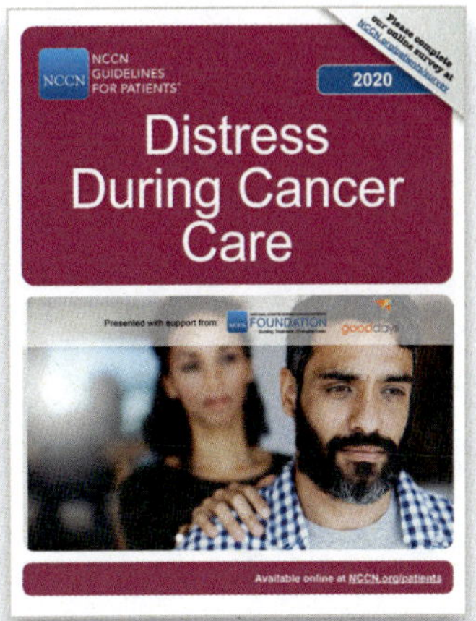

5

Second-line therapy

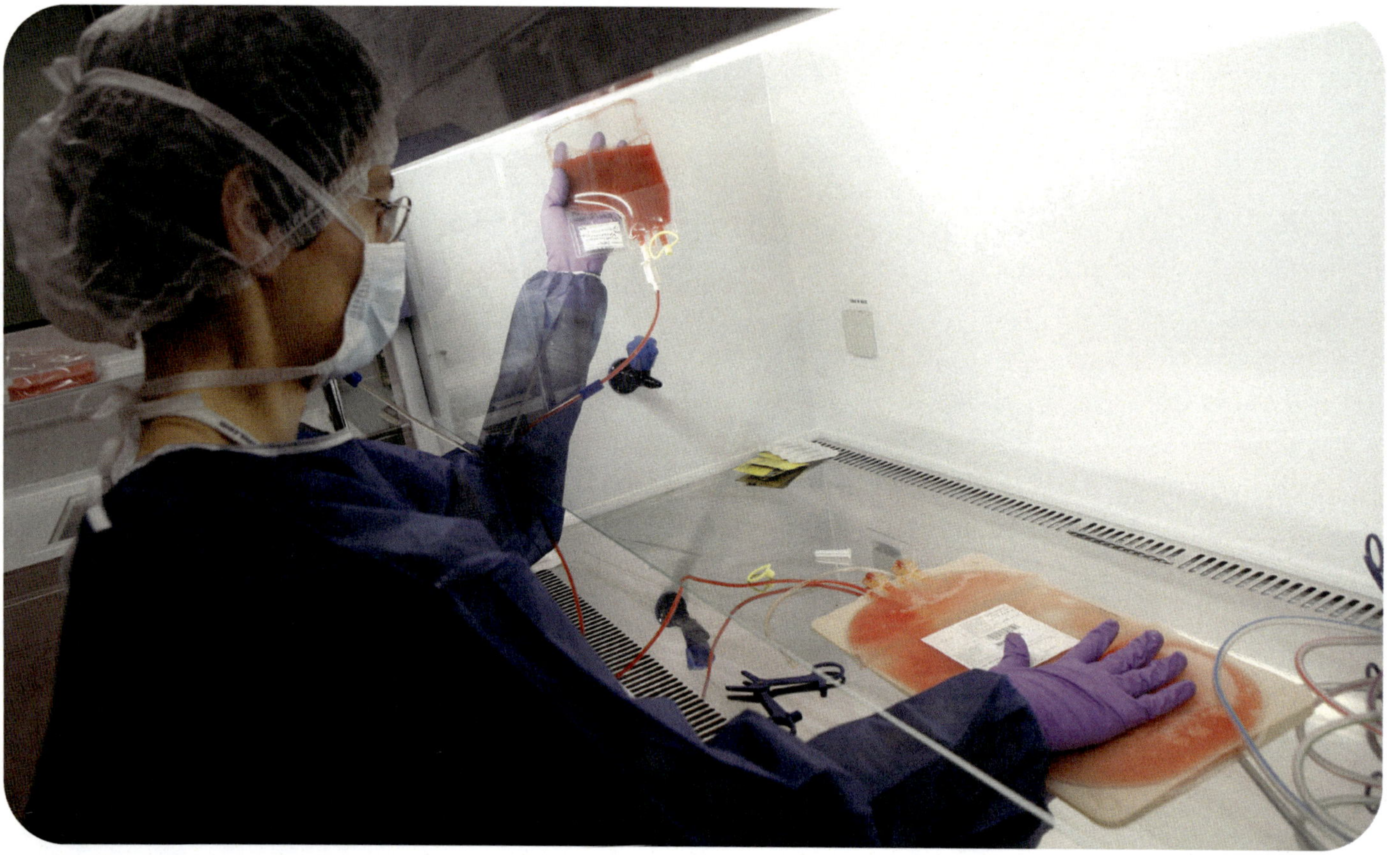

Peripheral T-cell lymphoma may come back after the first line of treatment. The goal of second-line treatment is to stop it from getting worse and to keep it from coming back again.

After first-line treatment, a lymphoma may not get better. It may even get worse. This is called refractory disease—it means the cancer didn't respond to treatment.

On the other hand, cancer may get better or even be in remission after treatment, but then come back again. This is called a relapse or recurrence. In many people, peripheral T-cell lymphoma often improves with treatment but eventually relapses.

The treatment for refractory and relapsed lymphoma is second-line therapy.

Second-line therapy

The goal of second-line therapy is to achieve remission. Remission is when some or all of the signs and symptoms of cancer have disappeared.

Second-line therapy options for peripheral T-cell lymphoma include:

- Clinical trial
- Single agents
- Combination chemotherapy
- Radiation therapy (palliative)
- Supportive care
- Observation

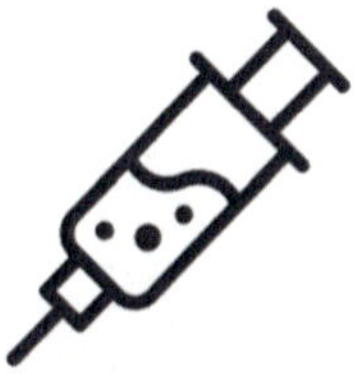

Stem cell transplant: To proceed or not to proceed?

A clinical trial is the preferred treatment option for relapsed or refractory peripheral T-cell lymphoma. But the choice of second-line therapy is also based on whether or not a patient is eligible for a stem cell transplant.

A stem cell transplant is a procedure that replaces damaged or destroyed stem cells with healthy stem cells. The healthy stem cells help to grow new blood cells.

A stem cell transplant is an intense treatment. It's not for everyone. It tends to be more successful in people who've had a complete or partial response to chemotherapy. A stem cell transplant is usually performed after second-line therapy is completed. (For more information about stem cell transplants, see Chapter 6.)

For patients with relapsed or refractory peripheral T-cell lymphoma who are ineligible for a stem cell transplant, the goal is to keep them in remission for as long as possible while maintaining their quality of life. Quality of life involves a person's overall enjoyment of life, including their sense of well-being and ability to participate in regular activities.

Second-line therapy for peripheral T-cell lymphoma

Stem cell transplant is planned

Second-line therapy options:

- Clinical trial (preferred)
- Single-agent or combination chemotherapy

Complete or partial response to therapy → Consolidation or additional therapy

No response to therapy or cancer worsens → Follow-up care

No stem cell transplant is planned

Second-line therapy options:

- Clinical trial (preferred)
- Single-agent or combination chemotherapy
- Palliative radiation therapy
- Supportive care

Response to therapy or clinical benefit → Continue treatment or be under observation

No response to therapy or cancer worsens → Follow-up care

Clinical trial

The preferred treatment option for all patients with relapsed or refractory peripheral T-cell lymphoma is a clinical trial. Clinical trials give people access to treatment options that they couldn't usually receive otherwise.

A clinical trial is not a "last ditch" treatment. It's considered a first-line therapy in many people with peripheral T-cell lymphoma. An NCCN panel of lymphoma experts strongly encourages people with relapsed or refractory peripheral T-cell lymphoma to enroll in a clinical trial if one is open and is the right fit.

Single agents

If a clinical trial isn't available or isn't the right choice, then second-line therapy for peripheral T-cell lymphoma involves chemotherapy.

But what type of chemotherapy? And should it be a combination of chemotherapy drugs or a single drug (also called a single agent)?

The choice of combination chemotherapy or a single agent should be based on factors like your age, physical ability (performance status), the type of T-cell lymphoma, the potential drug side effects, and the goals of therapy.

Single agents are useful for some people because they're simple to take, cause fewer or less harsh side effects, and still reduce symptoms. Newer single agent drugs may be more tolerable and equally effective as combination chemotherapy. Talk to your doctor about the different options and their risks and benefits.

Preferred single-agent drugs include:

Belinostat

Belinostat can be used as a single agent for second-line therapy. It's only for patients with relapsed or refractory peripheral T-cell lymphoma. It's given by IV infusion into a vein.

Brentuximab vedotin

Brentuximab vedotin is a drug conjugate that combines two drugs in one medicine (so it's still considered a single agent for second-line therapy). Brentuximab vedotin specifically targets cancer cells that have the CD30 protein. So it's only given to patients whose lab results show cancer cells with the CD30 protein.

Pralatrexate

Pralatrexate is a type of drug called a folate analogue metabolic inhibitor. The drug works by blocking (inhibiting) cancer cells from using folate, an essential B vitamin. Without folate, cancer cells can't multiply. Pralatrexate is only for patients with relapsed or refractory peripheral T-cell lymphoma. It's given by IV infusion once a week for 6 weeks. After a 1-week break, the cycle is started over again.

Romidepsin

Romidepsin is a single-agent drug that shuts down histones. Histones are proteins that are necessary for the formation of DNA in cancer cells. Without histones, cancer cells can die. Romidepsin is an IV infusion given once a week for 3 weeks followed by a 1-week break.

All single-agent drugs have side effects such as nausea, vomiting, diarrhea, tiredness, infection, fever, loss of appetite, and others.

Other recommended single-agents:

- Alemtuzumab
- Bendamustine
- Bortezomib
- Crizotinib (for ALK+ ALCL only)
- Cyclophosphamide and/or etoposide
- Cyclosporine (for AITL only)
- Gemcitabine
- Lenalidomide

Combination chemotherapy

For second-line therapy, a combination of drugs may be a better choice than a single agent for certain patients. These may be people who are comparatively younger, have good or adequate physical ability, or can handle a more difficult treatment regimen.

Combination chemo may also be appropriate in people who are eligible for a stem cell transplant after second-line therapy.

Second-line combination chemotherapy usually includes drugs that are different from those used in first-line chemotherapy. Some of these are platinum-based chemotherapy drugs (cisplatin, oxaliplatin, and carboplatin). These drugs disrupt DNA inside cancer cells, which causes the cells to die. Platinum-based chemotherapies are effective, but they can cause severe side effects. Also, cancer tends to quickly develop resistance to these drugs. **See Guide 4**.

Combination chemotherapy

...is when a few chemotherapy drugs are given at the same time.

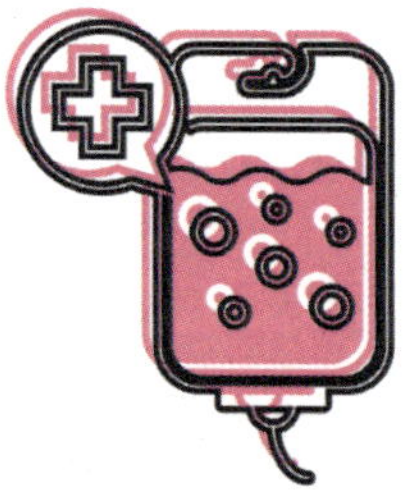

Combination chemotherapy can include drugs given as an intravenous (IV) infusion

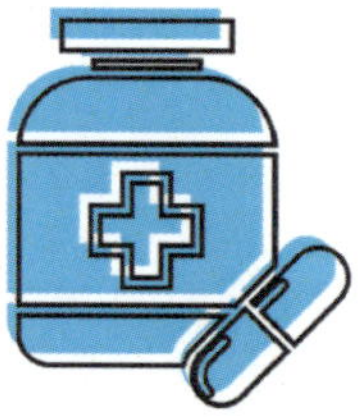

...and pills that you swallow.

Guide 4. Recommended second-line chemotherapy combinations for treating peripheral T-cell lymphoma

Chemotherapy combination	Abbreviation
• dexamethasone • cytarabine • cisplatin	DHAP
• dexamethasone • cytarabine • oxaliplatin	DHAX
• etoposide • methylprednisolone • cytarabine • platinum chemotherapy (cisplatin or oxaliplatin)	ESHAP
• gemcitabine • dexamethasone • cisplatin	GDP
• gemcitabine • oxaliplatin	GemOx
• gemcitabine • vinorelbine • liposomal doxorubicin	GVD
• ifosfamide • carboplatin • etoposide	ICE

These regimens are listed in alphabetical order, not in order of importance.

Palliative radiation therapy

Palliative means relieving symptoms that are caused by the cancer or other treatment-related side effects. Palliative therapy is meant to improve quality of life.

The purpose of palliative radiation therapy is to reduce cancer symptoms like pain or bleeding, and prevent symptoms from occurring. Palliative radiation therapy targets cancer cells only in a certain area of the body. This means that lower doses of radiation can be used and the treatment cycle can be shorter.

Supportive care

Supportive care aims to improve quality of life. It includes care for health issues caused by cancer and cancer treatment. Supportive care (also called palliative care) is important at any stage of cancer, not just at the end of life.

Supportive care addresses many needs. It can help with making treatment decisions. It can also assist with coordinating care between health providers. Notably, supportive care can help prevent or treat physical and emotional symptoms.

Of course, supportive care can also help with spiritual support, advance care planning (which means deciding what you would want if you become too sick to make medical decisions for yourself), and end-of-life concerns.

Treatment response

What happens after second-line therapy? Your doctors and treatment team—with your input—will make that decision based on how your lymphoma has responded to treatment.

Importantly, the next phase of therapy depends on whether a stem cell transplant is a goal of your treatment plan:

Stem cell transplant:

- **Complete response or partial response**
  Treatment options for people who have a complete or partial response to second-line therapy include a clinical trial or a stem cell transplant. For more information about stem cell transplants, turn to Chapter 6.
- **No response or progressive disease**
  People who have no response or progressive disease will move on to the next line of therapy or follow-up care.

No stem cell transplant:

- **Complete response or partial response**
  People who have a complete response or a partial response, and who aren't having a stem cell transplant, may continue with their current treatment or be under observation.
- **No response or progressive disease**
  People who have no response or progressive disease will move on to the next line of therapy or follow-up care. Sometimes a person's T-cell lymphoma doesn't respond to one treatment but responds very well to another.

Follow-up care

Follow-up occurs after completing treatment. The goal of follow-up care is to watch out for the cancer to come back or to get worse. During follow-up, you'll have regular visits with your doctor or oncologist.

Here's the usual follow-up schedule for peripheral T-cell lymphoma:

- **Every 3 to 6 months** – Doctor's visit for a clinical history and physical exam.
- **Every 6 to 12 months** – PET or PET/CT imaging for cancer surveillance

If any symptoms return, don't wait until your next visit. Contact your doctor.

In rare cases, a person's lymphoma returns but grows at a slow pace and doesn't cause any symptoms. Observation may be an option in these patients, particularly those who aren't expected to have a stem cell transplant. Observation means your doctors will watch for cancer growth with regular follow-up tests over a period of time. No treatment is given unless symptoms appear or your condition changes.

If symptoms come back or your condition changes during follow-up, you may need further treatment. For more information about further treatment, see Chapter 6.

Key points

- Second-line therapy is the treatment for refractory and relapsed lymphoma. Its goal is to achieve remission.
- The choice of second-line therapy is based on whether or not a patient is eligible for a stem cell transplant.
- The preferred treatment option for relapsed or refractory peripheral T-cell lymphoma is a clinical trial.
- A stem cell transplant uses chemotherapy to destroy cells in the bone marrow, which are replaced with healthy stem cells.
- The choice of using a single agent or combination chemotherapy for second-line therapy is based on factors like the patient's age, performance status, drug side effects, and the goals of therapy.
- Second-line combination chemotherapy may include platinum-based drugs.
- Palliative radiation therapy is for reducing cancer symptoms and preventing symptoms from occurring.
- Supportive care aims to improve quality of life. It's important at any stage of cancer, not just at the end of life.
- Observation means your doctors will test you regularly for cancer growth. You won't receive treatment unless something changes.

6 Consolidation and additional therapy

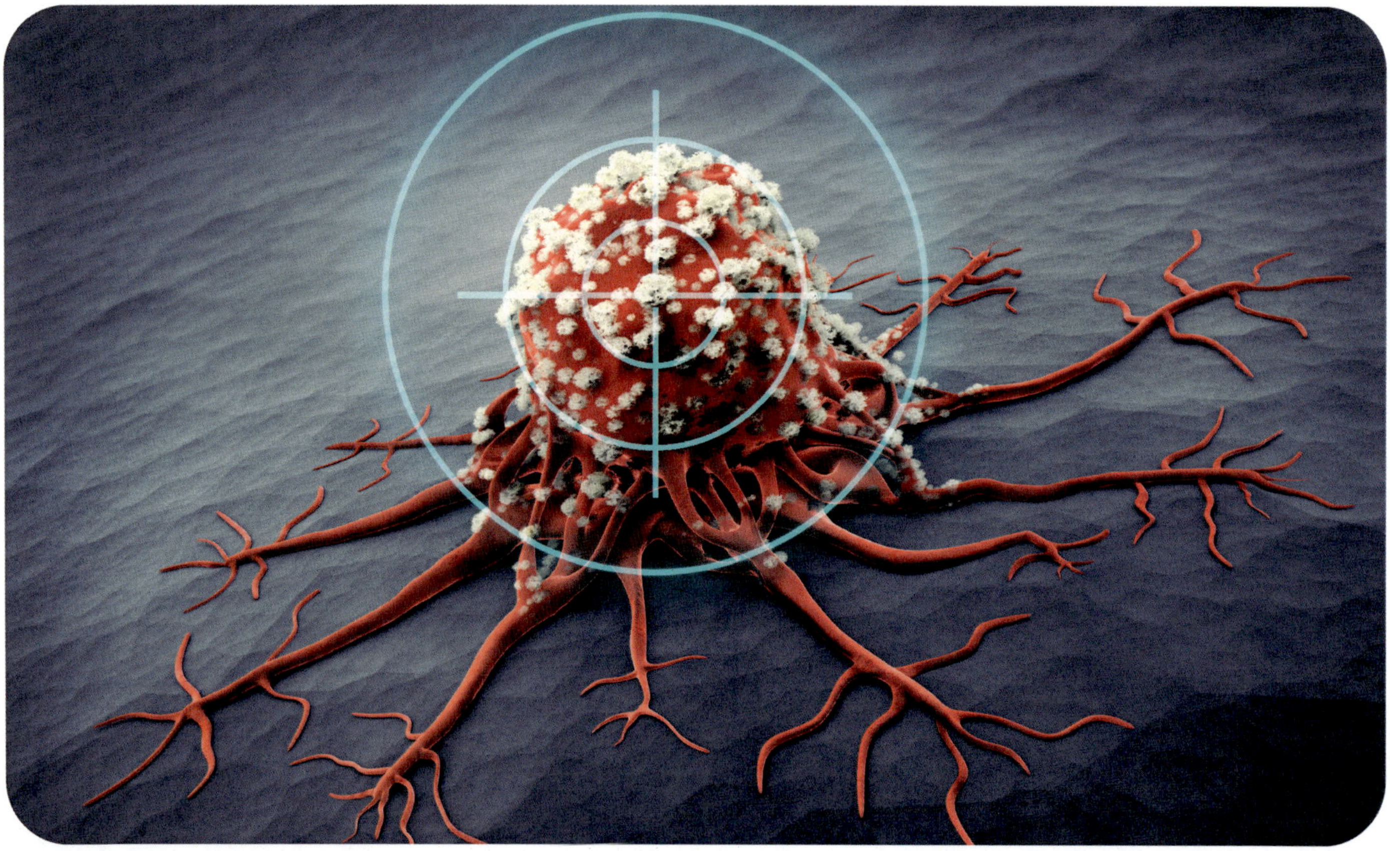

Consolidation and additional therapy are used to "clean up" any cancer left behind after first- or second-line therapies. A stem cell transplant can be a key part of this stage of therapy.

People with peripheral T-cell lymphoma who've had a partial or complete response to therapy—that is, when their signs and symptoms of lymphoma have decreased or disappeared—may be eligible to have consolidation therapy and additional therapy.

The purpose of consolidation therapy is to "clean up" any cancer cells that are left behind after first-line or second-line therapy. The goal is to prevent or delay the lymphoma from coming back.

Consolidation therapy and additional therapy options for peripheral T-cell lymphoma include:

- Clinical trial
- Stem cell transplant

Clinical trial

The recommended treatment option for consolidation is a clinical trial. Clinical trials give people access to treatment options that they couldn't usually receive otherwise.

A clinical trial is not a "last ditch" treatment. It's considered a first-line therapy in many people with peripheral T-cell lymphoma. For more information about clinical trials, see Chapter 4.

Stem cell transplant

A stem cell is a basic cell that develops into other types of cells. Blood stem cells are made in the bone marrow and make blood cells. But cancer and its treatment—especially when used in high doses—can damage and destroy cells in the bone marrow. A stem cell transplant (also called a bone marrow transplant) is a way to kickstart the bone marrow to make more healthy blood cells.

A stem cell transplant starts with chemotherapy that destroys cells in the bone marrow. These cells are replaced with healthy stem cells. The healthy stem cells grow bone marrow and new blood cells. A stem cell transplant is performed after other treatments (first- or second-line therapy) have already been given.

A stem cell transplant can be an intense procedure. Doctors consider many factors when deciding who will benefit from this treatment. Some of these factors include your fitness level, health status, organ function, cancer stage, previous treatments, other medical conditions, available supportive care, and additional factors—including your goals and preferences.

There are two types of stem cell transplants:

- **Autologous transplant** - An autologous stem cell transplant uses your own blood stem cells to regrow bone marrow. It's also called high-dose therapy with autologous stem cell rescue (HDT/ASCR). First, some of your healthy stem cells will be removed from your bone marrow or peripheral blood. Next, you'll receive intensive chemotherapy to kill the cancer cells in your body. It will also kill the blood-producing cells in your bone marrow. Lastly, your healthy stem cells will be infused (no surgery) into your body to "rescue" your bone marrow.
- **Allogeneic transplant** - An allogeneic transplant uses healthy stem cells from another person (donor). First, you'll receive treatment called conditioning to kill your bone marrow cells. Next, you'll receive an infusion of donor cells. These cells will form new, healthy bone marrow, which will make healthy red and white blood cells. They'll also attack cancer cells that weren't killed by earlier treatment.

Autologous transplant is sometimes chosen after first-line therapy, while allogeneic stem cell transplant is often recommended after second-line therapy. For people with refractory

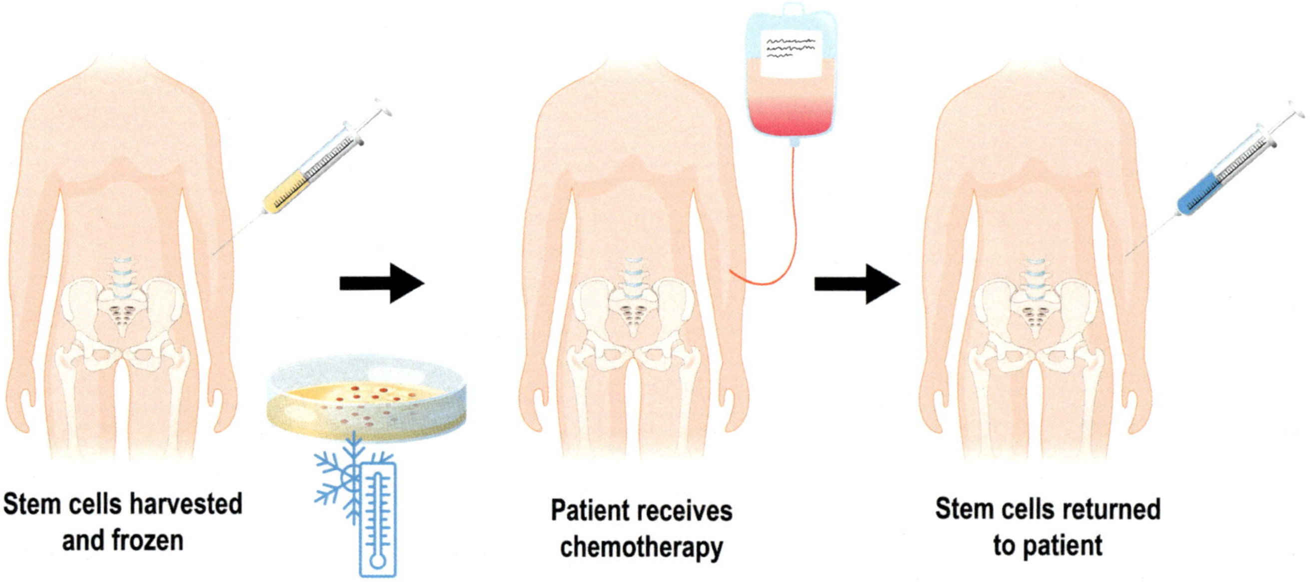

Autologous stem cell transplant

First, stem cells are removed ("harvested") from the patient's blood or bone marrow. Second, the harvested stem cells are concentrated and frozen for preservation. Meanwhile, the patient receives high-dose chemotherapy to destroy any cancer cells in the bone marrow. Lastly, the stem cells are returned ("transfused") to the patient, where they'll grow healthy new cells in the bone marrow.

or relapsed peripheral T-cell lymphoma, allogeneic stem cell transplant can be more effective but also more risky than an autologous stem cell transplant.

In some cases, radiation therapy can be used on specific (local) areas of lymphoma before or after high-dose chemotherapy.

A type of allogeneic transplant that involves less chemotherapy is called a reduced intensity transplant. This type of transplant relies on the donor cells' ability to attack and destroy cancer cells. A reduced intensity transplant is used more often in older patients and those who can't tolerate intense chemotherapy.

Side effects of stem cell transplant

High-dose chemotherapy can result in nausea, vomiting, diarrhea, hair loss, and mouth sores. You'll likely feel tired and weak after the transplant and while waiting for the new blood stem cells to grow in the bone marrow. This weak and unpleasant feeling might last for several weeks after you go home, too.

Also, you'll have to be extra careful to avoid germs in the first few weeks after the procedure because your infection-fighting immune system will be almost gone.

To learn more about stem cell transplants, visit the National Marrow Donor Program website at bethematch.org.

Follow-up care

Follow-up occurs after completing treatment. The goal of follow-up care is to watch out for the cancer to come back or to get worse. During follow-up, you'll have regular visits with your doctor or oncologist.

Here's the usual follow-up schedule for peripheral T-cell lymphoma:

- **Every 3 to 6 months** – Doctor's visit for a clinical history and physical exam.
- **Every 6 to 12 months** – PET or PET/CT imaging for cancer surveillance

If any symptoms return (recurrence), don't wait until your next visit. Contact your doctor right away. For more information about relapse, see Chapter 5.

Treatment doesn't necessarily end after second-line therapy. If symptoms come back or your condition changes during follow-up, you can try more treatment. Treatment may continue, off and on, for the rest of your life.

This can include one or more of the following options:

- Clinical trial
- Another second-line therapy
- Palliative radiation therapy
- Supportive care

After this treatment is completed, you'll either be observed or move on to the next treatment.

Key points

- Consolidation therapy is used to "clean up" any cancer cells left behind after first- or second-line therapy.
- There are two types of stem cell transplants used for consolidation:
  - An autologous stem cell transplant uses your own blood stem cells to regrow bone marrow.
  - An allogeneic transplant uses healthy stem cells from a donor.
- An allogeneic stem cell transplant can be more effective but also more risky than an autologous stem cell transplant for people with peripheral T-cell lymphoma.
- Follow-up care comes after completing treatment. The goal is to watch out for the cancer to come back or to get worse.
- Treatment doesn't necessarily end after first-line or second-line therapy. It may continue, off and on, for the rest of your life.

We want your feedback!

Our goal is to provide helpful and easy-to-understand information on cancer.

Take our survey to let us know what we got right and what we could do better:

NCCN.org/patients/feedback

7 Making treatment decisions

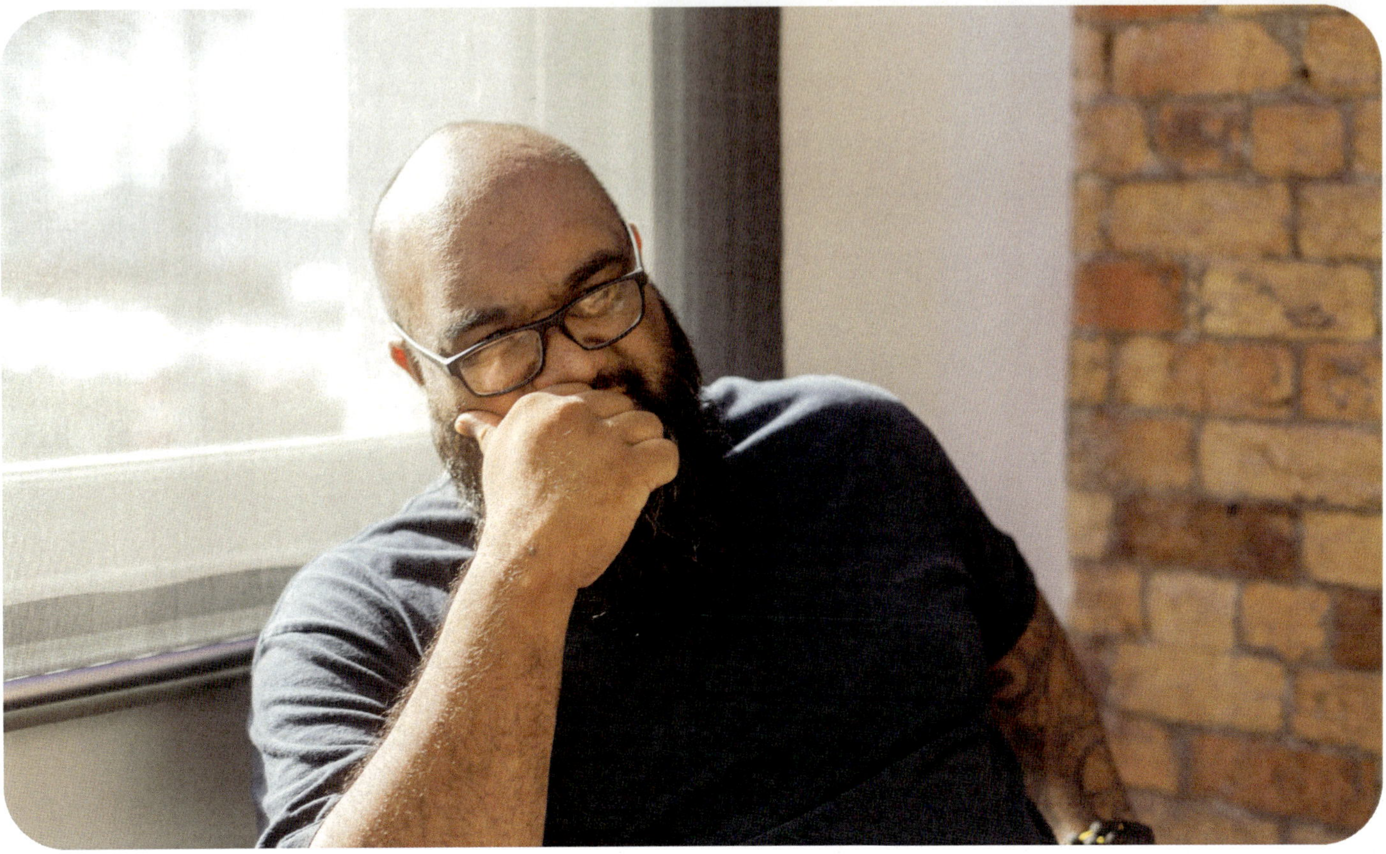

It's important to be comfortable with the treatment you choose. This choice starts with having an open and honest conversation with your doctors.

It's your choice

In shared decision-making, you and your doctors share information, discuss the options, and agree on a treatment plan. It starts with an open and honest conversation between you and your doctor.

Treatment decisions are very personal. What's important to you may not be important to someone else.

Some things that may play a role in your decision-making:

- What you want and how that might differ from what others want
- Availability of clinical trials in your area
- Your religious and spiritual beliefs
- Your feelings about certain treatments like chemotherapy or stem cell therapy
- Your feelings about pain or side effects such as nausea and vomiting
- Cost of treatment, travel to treatment centers, and time away from work
- Quality of life and length of life
- How active you are and the activities that are important to you

Think about what you want from treatment. Discuss openly the risks and benefits of specific treatments and procedures. Weigh options and share concerns with your doctor. If you make the effort to build a relationship with your doctor, it will help you feel supported when considering options and making treatment decisions. Learning about lymphoma will help you make better treatment decisions as you talk with your doctor.

Deciding on your treatment options

Choosing your treatment is a very important decision. It can affect your length and quality of life. But deciding which treatment option is best can be hard. Doctors from different fields of medicine may have different opinions on which option is best for you. This can be very confusing. Also, your spouse, partner, or family members may disagree with which option you want. That can be stressful. In some cases, one option hasn't been shown to work better than another.

Here are some ways to help you decide on treatment.

Second opinion

People with cancer often want to get treated as soon as possible. They want to make their cancer go away before it grows any further. While cancer can't be ignored, there is usually enough time to think about and choose which option is best for you.

You may completely trust your doctor, but a second opinion about which option is best can help. A second opinion is when another doctor reviews your test results and suggests a treatment plan. Copies of the pathology report, imaging, and other test results need to be sent to the doctor giving the second opinion. Some people feel uneasy asking for copies from their doctors. However, a second opinion is a normal part of cancer care and most doctors are very comfortable helping you to get a second opinion. Even doctors get second opinions!

Some health plans require a second opinion. If your health plan doesn't cover the cost of a second opinion, you have the choice of paying for it yourself.

If the two opinions are the same, you may feel more at peace about treatment. If the two opinions differ, think about getting a third opinion. A third opinion may help you decide between your options. It's your cancer, and the decision about which treatment is best is your decision.

Things you can do to prepare for a second opinion:

- Check with your insurance company about its rules on second opinions. There may be out-of-pocket costs to see doctors who aren't part of your insurance plan.
- Make plans to have copies of all your records sent to the doctor you will see for your second opinion.

Compare benefits and downsides

Every option has benefits and downsides. Consider both when deciding which option is best for you. Talking to others can help identify benefits and downsides you haven't thought of. Scoring each factor from 0 to 10 can also help because some factors may be more important to you than others.

Get group support

Many people with cancer find a lot of value in a support group. In support groups, you can ask questions and hear about the experiences of other people with cancer. Some people may be newly diagnosed, while others may be finished with treatment.

A support group can help with emotional and psychological needs. A support group can also be a good source of practical advice and helpful tips. People with common ground can share information on their experiences, financial and emotional burdens, coping strategies, and knowledge about research and treatments.

Ask your doctors or supportive care team about finding a lymphoma or cancer support community. Support groups can be found online and in-person groups are often available in larger communities.

Questions to ask your doctors

Possible questions to ask your doctors are listed on the following pages. Feel free to use these questions or come up with your own. Be clear about your goals for treatment and find out what to expect from treatment.

Questions to ask about testing and staging

1. What type of lymphoma do I have?
2. Can this cancer be cured? If not, how well can treatment stop it from growing?
3. What tests will I have?
4. Will I have more than one biopsy?
5. How do I prepare for testing?
6. What if I'm pregnant or planning to get pregnant?
7. Where do I go to get tested? How long will the tests take? Will any test hurt?
8. How often are these tests wrong?
9. Should I bring someone with me?
10. Should I bring a list of my medications?
11. How soon will I know the results and who will explain them to me?
12. Would you give me a copy of the pathology report and other test results?
13. Will my biopsy tissue be saved for further testing? Can I have it sent to another facility for additional testing?
14. Who will talk with me about the next steps? When?
15. Who can I call if I need help immediately?
16. Can I get a second opinion? Who would you recommend I see for a second opinion?

Questions to ask about treatment options

1. What are my treatment options? Are you suggesting options from the NCCN Guidelines, or have you modified the standard approach in my situation?
2. How many patients like me have you treated?
3. Will the treatment hurt?
4. What will happen if I do nothing?
5. How do my age, overall health, and other factors affect my options?
6. Does any option offer a cure or long-term cancer control? Are my chances any better for one option than another? Less time-consuming? Less expensive?
7. Do your suggested options include clinical trials? Please explain why.
8. How do you know if my treatment is working?
9. How will I know if my treatment is working, and how long does it usually take?
10. What are my options if treatment stops working?
11. What are the possible complications? What are the short- and long-term side effects of treatment?
12. How will treatment affect me? Will my sense of smell or taste change? Will my hair fall out?
13. How soon will I need to make my treatment decisions?
14. What can be done to prevent or relieve the side effects of treatment?
15. What supportive care services are available to me during and after treatment?
16. Can I stop treatment at any time? What will happen if I stop treatment?

Questions to ask about getting treatment

1. Do I have to go to the hospital or elsewhere? How often? How long is each visit?
2. What do I need to think about if I will travel for treatment?
3. Do I have a choice of when to begin treatment? Can I choose the days and times of treatment?
4. How do I prepare for treatment? Do I have to stop taking any of my medicines? Are there foods I should avoid?
5. Should I bring someone with me when I get treated?
6. How much will the treatment cost me? What does my insurance cover? Are there any grants available to me?
7. Will I miss work or school? Will I be able to drive?
8. What should I do on weekends or non-office hours if I have an urgent problem with my cancer or my cancer treatment? Who do I call when you're off duty? Should I go to the emergency room?
9. Is home care after treatment needed? If yes, what type?
10. Will I be able to manage my own health?
11. Will I be able to return to my normal activities? If so, when?
12. What emotional and psychological help is available for me and those taking care of me?

Questions to ask about clinical trials

1. Are there clinical trials for my type of lymphoma?
2. What are the treatments used in the clinical trial?
3. What does the treatment do?
4. Has the treatment been used before? Has it been used for other types of cancer?
5. What are the risks and benefits of joining the clinical trial and the treatment being tested?
6. Will the trial need a biopsy sample?
7. What side effects should I expect? How will the side effects be controlled?
8. How long will I be in the clinical trial?
9. Will I be able to get other treatment if this doesn't work?
10. How will you know if the treatment is working?
11. Will the clinical trial cost me anything? If so, how much?

Online resources

American Cancer Society
cancer.org/cancer/non-hodgkin-lymphoma.html

Blood & Marrow Transplant Information Network (BMT InfoNet)
bmtinfonet.org

Leukemia & Lymphoma Society
www.lls.org/lymphoma

Lymphoma Research Foundation
lymphoma.org/aboutlymphoma/nhl/

MedlinePlus
medlineplus.gov/lymphoma.html

National Bone Marrow Transplant Link (nbmtLINK)
nbmtlink.org

National Marrow Donor Program
bethematch.org

National Cancer Institute
cancer.gov/types/lymphoma

National Coalition for Cancer Survivorship
canceradvocacy.org

NCCN Patient and Caregiver Resources
NCCN.org/patientresources/patient-resources/support-for-patients-caregivers

share with us.

Take our survey
And help make the NCCN Guidelines for Patients better for everyone!

NCCN.org/patients/comments

Words to know

advance care planning
The process of deciding what you would want if you become too sick to make medical decisions for yourself.

allogenic stem cell transplant
A cancer treatment that destroys cells in the bone marrow and replaces them with healthy stem cells from a donor.

autologous stem cell transplant
A cancer treatment that destroys cells in the bone marrow and replaces them with your own healthy stem cells.

B symptoms
A set of symptoms (fever, night sweats, weight loss) that may indicate a widespread or advanced lymphoma.

biopsy
A procedure that removes tissue or fluid samples to be tested for disease.

bone marrow
A soft, spongy material inside of bones where most blood cells are made.

chemotherapy
Cancer drugs that stop the cell life cycle so cells don't increase in number.

clinical trial
A type of research that assesses investigational tests or treatments in people.

combination chemotherapy
Treatment that combines two or more chemotherapy drugs. Also called multi-agent chemotherapy.

diagnosis
The identification of an illness based on tests.

first-line therapy
The first type of treatment given for a condition or disease. First-line therapy is the one considered to be the best treatment.

follow-up care
Health care that starts once treatment has ended and there are no signs of cancer.

gastrointestinal (GI) tract
The group of organs (including the stomach, intestines, and others) through which food passes after being eaten.

extranodal disease
Lymphoma that occurs in areas of the body other than the lymph nodes.

hematopathologist
A doctor who diagnoses diseases of blood cells.

immune system
The body's natural defense against infection and disease.

immunophenotyping
A lab test that identifies cells based on the particular proteins on the cells' surface.

lymph
A clear fluid containing infection-fighting white blood cells. Lymph also gives cells water and food.

lymph node
A small, bean-shaped, disease-fighting structure in the immune system.

lymphatic system
A network of organs and vessels that fights infections and transports a fluid called lymph.

lymphocyte
One of three main types of white blood cells that help protect the body from infection.

lymphoma
A cancer that begins in white blood cells (lymphocytes) within the lymphatic system.

observation
A period of watching for cancer growth or occurrence while not receiving treatment.

palliative therapy
Health care that includes symptom relief but not cancer treatment. Also sometimes called supportive care.

performance status
A rating of a person's ability to do daily activities.

positron emission tomography and computed tomography (PET/CT) scan
An imaging test that uses two picture-making methods to show the shape and function of organs and tissues inside the body.

prognosis
The likely course and outcome of a disease based on tests and response to treatment.

progression
A cancer that is spreading, growing, or getting worse.

radiation therapy
A treatment that uses high-energy rays (radiation) to kill cancer cells.

refractory cancer
A cancer that doesn't improve with treatment.

relapse
The return or worsening of cancer after a period of improvement.

remission
The absence of cancer signs and symptoms after treatment.

restaging
The process of rating the extent of cancer in the body after therapy.

second-line therapy
The second type of treatment given if the first treatment doesn't work or stops working.

side effect
An unhealthy or unpleasant physical or emotional response to treatment.

staging
The process of rating the extent of cancer in the body.

stem cell transplant
A cancer treatment that uses chemotherapy to destroy cells in the bone marrow, which are replaced with healthy blood stem cells.

supportive care
Health care for the symptoms of cancer or for the side effects of cancer treatment. Also sometimes called palliative care.

symptom
A feeling or problem that can indicate a disease or condition.

T cell
A type of white blood cell (lymphocyte) that defends against infection.

NCCN Contributors

This patient guide is based on the NCCN Clinical Practice Guidelines in Oncology (NCCN Guidelines®) for T-Cell Lymphomas, Version 1.2022. It was adapted, reviewed, and published with help from the following people:

Dorothy A. Shead, MS
Senior Director
Patient Information Operations

John Murphy
Medical Writer

Susan Kidney
Senior Graphic Design Specialist

The NCCN Clinical Practice Guidelines in Oncology (NCCN Guidelines®) for T-Cell Lymphomas, Version 1.2022 were developed by the following NCCN Panel Members:

Steven M. Horwitz, MD/Chair
Memorial Sloan Kettering Cancer Center

Stephen Ansell, MD, PhD/Vice-Chair
Mayo Clinic Cancer Center

Weiyun Z. Ai, MD, PhD
UCSF Helen Diller Family Comprehensive Cancer Center

Jeffrey Barnes, MD, PhD
Massachusetts General Hospital Cancer Center

*Stefan K. Barta, MD, MRCP, MS
Abramson Cancer Center at the University of Pennsylvania

*Jonathan Brammer, MD
The Ohio State University Comprehensive Cancer Center - James Cancer Hospital and Solove Research Institute

Mark W. Clemens, MD
The University of Texas MD Anderson Cancer Center

Ahmet Dogan, MD, PhD
Memorial Sloan Kettering Cancer Center

Francine Foss, MD
Yale Cancer Center/Smilow Cancer Hospital

Paola Ghione, MD
Roswell Park Comprehensive Cancer Center

Aaron M. Goodman, MD
UC San Diego Moores Cancer Center

Joan Guitart, MD
Robert H. Lurie Comprehensive Cancer Center of Northwestern University

Ahmad Halwani, MD
Huntsman Cancer Institute at the University of Utah

Bradley M. Haverkos, MD, MPH, MS
University of Colorado Cancer Center

Richard T. Hoppe, MD
Stanford Cancer Institute

Eric Jacobsen, MD
Dana-Farber/Brigham and Women's Cancer Center

*Deepa Jagadeesh, MD, MPH
Case Comprehensive Cancer Center/ University Hospitals Seidman Cancer Center and Cleveland Clinic Taussig Cancer Institute

Allison Jones, MD
St. Jude Children's Research Hospital/ The University of Tennessee Health Science Center

Avyakta Kallam, MD, MBBS
Fred & Pamela Buffett Cancer Center

Youn H. Kim, MD
Stanford Cancer Institute

Kiran Kumar, MD, MBA
UT Southwestern Simmons Comprehensive Cancer Center

Neha Mehta-Shah, MD, MSCI
Siteman Cancer Center at Barnes-Jewish Hospital and Washington University School of Medicine

Elise A. Olsen, MD
Duke Cancer Institute

Saurabh A. Rajguru, MD
University of Wisconsin Carbone Cancer Center

Sima Rozati, MD, PhD
The Sidney Kimmel Comprehensive Cancer Center at Johns Hopkins

Jonathan Said, MD
UCLA Jonsson Comprehensive Cancer Center

Aaron Shaver, MD, PhD
Vanderbilt-Ingram Cancer Center

*Lauren Shea, MD
O'Neal Comprehensive Cancer Center at UAB

Michi M. Shinohara, MD
Fred Hutchinson Cancer Research Center/ Seattle Cancer Care Alliance

Lubomir Sokol, MD, PhD
Moffitt Cancer Center

Carlos Torres-Cabala, MD
The University of Texas MD Anderson Cancer Center

Ryan Wilcox, MD, PhD
University of Michigan Rogel Cancer Center

Peggy Wu, MD, MPH
UC Davis Comprehensive Cancer Center

Jasmine Zain, MD
City of Hope National Medical Center

NCCN

Mary Dwyer, MS
Hema Sundar, PhD

* Reviewed this patient guide. For disclosures, visit NCCN.org/disclosures.

NCCN Cancer Centers

Abramson Cancer Center
at the University of Pennsylvania
Philadelphia, Pennsylvania
800.789.7366 • pennmedicine.org/cancer

Fred & Pamela Buffett Cancer Center
Omaha, Nebraska
402.559.5600 • unmc.edu/cancercenter

Case Comprehensive Cancer Center/
University Hospitals Seidman Cancer
Center and Cleveland Clinic Taussig
Cancer Institute
Cleveland, Ohio
800.641.2422 • UH Seidman Cancer Center
uhhospitals.org/services/cancer-services
866.223.8100 • CC Taussig Cancer Institute
my.clevelandclinic.org/departments/cancer
216.844.8797 • Case CCC
case.edu/cancer

City of Hope National Medical Center
Los Angeles, California
800.826.4673 • cityofhope.org

Dana-Farber/Brigham and
Women's Cancer Center |
Massachusetts General Hospital
Cancer Center
Boston, Massachusetts
617.732.5500
youhaveus.org
617.726.5130
massgeneral.org/cancer-center

Duke Cancer Institute
Durham, North Carolina
888.275.3853 • dukecancerinstitute.org

Fox Chase Cancer Center
Philadelphia, Pennsylvania
888.369.2427 • foxchase.org

Huntsman Cancer Institute
at the University of Utah
Salt Lake City, Utah
800.824.2073
huntsmancancer.org

Fred Hutchinson Cancer
Research Center/Seattle
Cancer Care Alliance
Seattle, Washington
206.606.7222 • seattlecca.org
206.667.5000 • fredhutch.org

The Sidney Kimmel Comprehensive
Cancer Center at Johns Hopkins
Baltimore, Maryland
410.955.8964
www.hopkinskimmelcancercenter.org

Robert H. Lurie Comprehensive Cancer
Center of Northwestern University
Chicago, Illinois
866.587.4322 • cancer.northwestern.edu

Mayo Clinic Cancer Center
Phoenix/Scottsdale, Arizona
Jacksonville, Florida
Rochester, Minnesota
480.301.8000 • Arizona
904.953.0853 • Florida
507.538.3270 • Minnesota
mayoclinic.org/cancercenter

Memorial Sloan Kettering
Cancer Center
New York, New York
800.525.2225 • mskcc.org

Moffitt Cancer Center
Tampa, Florida
888.663.3488 • moffitt.org

The Ohio State University
Comprehensive Cancer Center -
James Cancer Hospital and
Solove Research Institute
Columbus, Ohio
800.293.5066 • cancer.osu.edu

O'Neal Comprehensive
Cancer Center at UAB
Birmingham, Alabama
800.822.0933 • uab.edu/onealcancercenter

Roswell Park Comprehensive
Cancer Center
Buffalo, New York
877.275.7724 • roswellpark.org

Siteman Cancer Center at Barnes-
Jewish Hospital and Washington
University School of Medicine
St. Louis, Missouri
800.600.3606 • siteman.wustl.edu

St. Jude Children's Research Hospital/
The University of Tennessee
Health Science Center
Memphis, Tennessee
866.278.5833 • stjude.org
901.448.5500 • uthsc.edu

Stanford Cancer Institute
Stanford, California
877.668.7535 • cancer.stanford.edu

UC Davis
Comprehensive Cancer Center
Sacramento, California
916.734.5959 • 800.770.9261
health.ucdavis.edu/cancer

UC San Diego Moores Cancer Center
La Jolla, California
858.822.6100 • cancer.ucsd.edu

UCLA Jonsson
Comprehensive Cancer Center
Los Angeles, California
310.825.5268 • cancer.ucla.edu

UCSF Helen Diller Family
Comprehensive Cancer Center
San Francisco, California
800.689.8273 • cancer.ucsf.edu

University of Colorado Cancer Center
Aurora, Colorado
720.848.0300 • coloradocancercenter.org

University of Michigan
Rogel Cancer Center
Ann Arbor, Michigan
800.865.1125 • rogelcancercenter.org

The University of Texas
MD Anderson Cancer Center
Houston, Texas
844.269.5922 • mdanderson.org

University of Wisconsin
Carbone Cancer Center
Madison, Wisconsin
608.265.1700 • uwhealth.org/cancer

UT Southwestern Simmons
Comprehensive Cancer Center
Dallas, Texas
214.648.3111 • utsouthwestern.edu/simmons

Vanderbilt-Ingram Cancer Center
Nashville, Tennessee
877.936.8422 • vicc.org

Yale Cancer Center/
Smilow Cancer Hospital
New Haven, Connecticut
855.4.SMILOW • yalecancercenter.org

Index

Made in the USA
Monee, IL
22 April 2022

95142880R00043